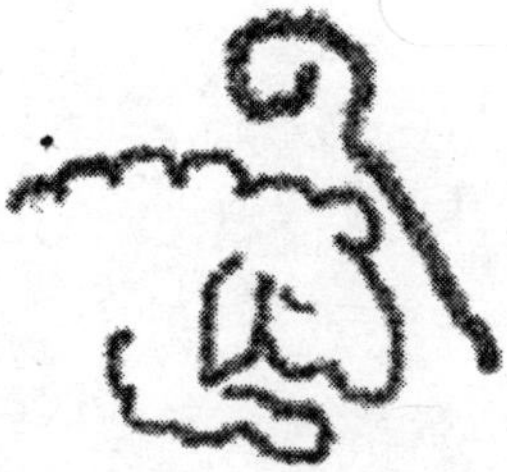

Effective Pastoral Counseling

Gary Collins

OMF LITERATURE INC.
PO BOX 2217 MANILA, PHILIPPINES

Effective Pastoral Counseling

The publishers are grateful to be able to use materials from:

Effective Counseling *by Gary Collins, copyright © 1972 by Creation House;*
Man in Transition *by Gary Collins, copyright © 1971 by Creation House;*
Fractured Personalities *by Gary Collins, copyright © 1972 by Creation House.*
Used with permission.

Overcoming Anxiety, *published and copyrighted by Vision House Publishers.*
Used with permission.

The publishers acknowledge the contribution of Dr. Russell G. Honeywell, Founder and former President of Febias College of Bible, who selected the material for inclusion in the first draft of Effective Pastoral Counseling.

Published (1984) by
OMF Literature Inc.
776 Boni Avenue
Mandaluyong City, Metro Manila

Reprinted — 1987, 1988, 1991, 1993, 1996
Revised edition — 1996
Reprinted — 1999, 2000 (new cover)

ISBN 971-511-417-2

Printed in the Philippines

Contents

Foreword

Almost ten years have passed since my first visit to South East Asia, but I still cherish the memory of that initial trip. My lectures on Christian counseling were received with a warmth and enthusiasm which has been repeated in country after country as God has given me the privilege of meeting with pastors and Christian friends - some of whom will never read this book.

During His brief time on earth, Jesus showed deep compassion for His fellow human beings. He instructed His disciples to comfort the sick and care for the needy. The early Christians, in His church, ministered to each other, and the New Testament writers instructed us to help, encourage, and build up one another. Bearing one another's burdens (Galatians 6:2) was shown to be a mark of Christian love, and believers were taught to "do good to all men," - especially to those who are fellow Christians.

Counseling, therefore, is not a new fad or a distinctly North American idea. Christian counseling is a biblical concept. It is based on the teachings of Scripture, and has been practiced in one form or another throughout church history. Counseling is not meant to replace preaching, teaching, or the discipling of believers. Instead, helping people is a vital part of the whole ministry of the church.

Of course, counseling occurs in many languages and it must be adapted both to the needs of the people seeking help and to the cultures in which we live. The principles which you read in the pages of this book are not meant to be applied rigidly. They are presented, instead, as guidelines to help you minister to the people in your community.

I am humbled and deeply gratified to see this book appear in print. It is my prayer that the Holy Spirit will use it to guide you into an effective counseling ministry.

Gary R. Collins

I

Basic Considerations in Counseling

1

Basic Considerations

When the children of Israel were camped at the foot of Mount Horeb, Moses had a visit from his father-in-law, a man named Jethro (Exodus 18:1-7). The older man was glad to learn details about the journey from Egypt, but he was distressed to discover that Moses was spending entire days listening to complaints and "judging" the people. Then, as in-laws are sometimes inclined to do, Jethro decided to offer advice. He told Moses that he was wearing himself out and suggested that "able men" be selected to handle some of the less serious problems. These men were to be God-fearing, honest (Exodus 18:21), available "at all times" (18:22 *RSV*), and willing to refer the more difficult problems to Moses (18:26).

Counseling can be defined as a relationship between two or more persons in which one person (the counselor) seeks to advise, encourage and/or assist another person or persons (the counselee/s) to deal more effectively with the problems of life. Counseling may have several goals, including changing the counselee's behavior, attitudes or values; preventing more serious problems from developing; teaching social skills; encouraging expression of emotions; giving support in times of need; instilling insight; guiding as a decision is made; teaching responsibility; stimulating spiritual growth; and helping the counselee to mobilize his inner resources in times of crisis. Unlike psychotherapy, counseling rarely aims to radically alter or remold the personality.

Because of his position, the church leader is in a unique counseling position. Unlike the professional, the pastoral counselor is often well-acquainted with the counselee's personal, home and community background. The church leader can visit in homes, he is often a trusted friend, and he is available. In addition, the pastoral counselor freely makes use of spiritual resources such as prayer and Bible reading. Since he strives to be an "expert in spiritual growth,"[1] the Christian counselor can be of special help to the people who are concerned about God, values, sin, forgiveness, guilt and other religious questions.

THE SETTING FOR COUNSELING

Counseling can be done almost anywhere - in a home, in the pastor's office, at the back of an empty church, or in a hospital room. Privacy is of importance, however, and for this reason it is best to find a quiet location where there will be a minimum of interruptions.

There can be no hard and fast rules about the way in which a counseling room is furnished. If the church leader has an office where he does most of his counseling it is good idea for him to sit in the counselee's chair for a few minutes and look around. Are you gazing into a bright light or facing a distracting picture? Is the chair comfortable? Do you have an unobstructed view of the counselor's chair? If the room is pleasantly furnished, the counselor and counselee are both likely to feel more relaxed and able to do a better job.

Sometimes it is forgotten that the counselor's behavior also contributes to the setting. If he is busy leafing through papers, doodling, or slouched in his chair, he gives the impression that he is bored or more interested in other things.

If we are sincerely interested in people and want to help, this will "come across" and will be one of our most valuable assets in getting the counseling off to a good start.

PERSONAL CHARACTERISTICS OF THE COUNSELOR

Self-understanding

Freud believed that as a first step in becoming competent, the counselor must develop "insight into the . . . unconscious layers of his own soul."[2] To achieve this goal, he recommended that all counselors be analyzed by a trained therapist. While this suggestion has been rejected by most modern psychologists, it is generally agreed that self-understanding is a very desirable counselor characteristic. By knowing about ourselves we are better able to evaluate and control our own behavior, and we can more fully appreciate the feelings and actions of our counselee.[3] "The counselor who has not faced up to the problems of his own life, his own methods of evasion and self-deception, his own rationalizations, will have little understanding of these devices as they are employed by others."[4]

Self-knowledge includes an awareness of our beliefs and values. What we believe influences all of our interpersonal relations – including counseling – so we might as well recognize and accept our biases and, at times, even tell the counselee about them.[5]

Self-knowledge can never be complete, but there are at least three ways in which we can come to know ourselves better. First is reflection when alone - taking a personal inventory of our characteristics, strengths and weaknesses. Secondly, after looking conscientiously and honestly at ourselves, it is helpful to discuss the results with a respected friend or an experienced counselor. Frequently he will see things that we fail to recognize in ourselves. Thirdly, there is the self-understanding that comes when we ask the Holy Spirit to guide the evaluation. The God of Creation knows more about us than we will ever know (Psalm 139:1-6). With the psalmist we can pray, "Search me, O God, and know my heart: try me, and know my thoughts: and see if there be any wicked way in me, and lead me in the way everlasting" (Psalm 139:23-24).

Psychological characteristics

Textbook writers have listed a number of psychological traits which are assumed to make counselors more effective, including sincerity, compassion, patience, flexibility, self-confidence, optimism, approachability, mental alertness, common sense, fairness, emotional stability, good grooming, freedom from distracting mannerisms, breadth of knowledge, and ability to keep from appearing shocked. While all are desirable and worth developing, it is unlikely that any one person could possess them all or that all are necessary for successful counseling.

Understanding of others If the relationship is to be fruitful, the counselor must have at least some understanding of the counselee. By listening carefully, watching the counselee's behavior during the interview, and attempting to see things from his perspective, we can increase our understanding of his feelings, attitudes, and problems. In so doing, we also demonstrate our own interest and concern.

Acceptance This involves genuine respect and interest in the counselee as a "person" rather than as a "case." Such acceptance does not necessarily mean approval or agreement, for we may not like a person's opinions and may conclude that his past behavior is repulsive or sinful. But we must accept him as a person whom God loves and for whom Christ died.

Social distance Counselors were once taught that they should be completely uninvolved and emotionally detached from their counselees, but today it is recognized that cold aloofness and close personal involvement are equally undesirable. The counselor must be sufficiently detached to be objective but sufficiently involved to "feel with" the counselee. Occasionally he may express his own emotions or share something from his personal experience.

Ability to get along with people Good counselors are at ease in a variety of social settings. If a person generally has trouble relating to people, this will not suddenly change in a counseling room. The key to success is "not so much the techniques employed, important as they are, rather it is the total attitude of the counselor, how he feels about people, what he believes about them and about himself."[6]

Experience Counselors with greater experience often show more self-confidence and an increased ability to understand, accept, and successfully help their counselees.[7]

Spiritual characteristics

The effective Christian counselor must also possess spiritual qualifications. First he must be a Christian, having personally experienced the new birth (John 3:3) by believing that the risen Christ is the Son of God (John 3:15-17; Romans 10:9). Then, as in the days of Moses, pastoral counselors should be capable, God-fearing, honest, readily available, and willing to get help when they encounter difficult cases (Exodus 18:21-22). The counselor should also be a student who is thoroughly familiar with the Word of God (2 Timothy 2:15), and a man who seeks to be a follower of Christ (1 Peter 2:21) whose very name is "Wonderful Counselor" (Isaiah 9:6, *RSV*).

CHARACTERISTICS OF THE COUNSELEE

Effective counseling is not completely dependent on the counselor's characteristics and skills. If the counselee is uncooperative or uninterested in changing his behavior, the interviews will not be very fruitful, regardless of the counselor's skills. When children are forced to "talk with the pastor," for example, or when rebellious delinquents are *sent* for psychiatric help, often there is little improvement. For best results, the counselee must really want to change.

COUNSELING SKILLS AND TECHNIQUES

Good counseling is difficult work. It is time-consuming, emotionally draining, physically exhausting and frequently unsuccessful. By developing proficiency in the following skills and techniques, however, we should be able to increase our overall counseling effectiveness.

Before the interview

Whenever possible, it is best to spend a few minutes in preparation prior to the start of a counseling session. When we receive guests into our houses, we usually tidy the house and give the appearance that the guest is welcome and expected. A person coming for counseling should be received with at least as much courtesy. If he feels that he is "taking the valuable time of a busy man" he may feel guilty, rushed, and hence unable to communicate. It is a good procedure, therefore, to straighten the papers on the desk, get the room in readiness, and arrange to keep the counseling period free from interruptions.

Then we should review the counselee's case history and remind ourselves of the details of any previous counseling with him. It is embarrassing to get one person's problem confused with another's, and it is distressing to the counselee, who naturally prefers to think that he and his problems are uppermost in your mind.

For the Christian counselor it is also important to prepare for the interview with prayer. We can commit the counseling session to God, asking that we will be made sensitive to the needs and feelings of the counselee, and that we will be led by the Holy Spirit as we counsel.[8] Such prayer is no substitute for training and preparation, but all our activities, including those for which we are highly trained, should be committed to the Lord who guides our thoughts and actions (Proverbs 16:3; 3:5-6). The counselor should meet the counselee at the exact time of appointment. Being ten or fifteen minutes late and giving no real explanation will make the counselee assume he has been forgotten or that he isn't important enough to meet on time.

During the interview

The counseling session must be primarily a relationship between concerned people rather than a period which the counselor is so concerned about skills that he forgets everything else.

Start by working on the relationship Counselees often approach an interview with fear, trembling, and a number of misconceptions. They may be uncomfortable at the thought of discussing their personal problems, and uncertain about what is going to happen during the interview. At the beginning, therefore, the counselor has a responsibility to support and stimulate the counselee.[9] *Support* involves "breaking the ice" with a casual comment or two and inviting the counselee to have a seat. With some counselees it might be desirable to give an indication of what will happen during the interview. For example, the counselor might say, "I'm glad for this opportunity to chat about the things that are concerning you." This is much less threatening than an emotionally loaded statement like "I'm glad for this chance to counsel you about your problems."

(When someone brings a problem to a psychologist, the initial contact is usually a meeting between two strangers. In pastoral counseling, the counselor and counselee often know each other at least casually. Casual pre-counseling experiences do a great deal to establish a relationship long before the counselee ever knocks at your door.)

In addition to giving support and helping the person feel more at ease, we must *stimulate* him to talk. For some counselees this is no problem because they talk freely when given the chance. But, for others, talking is difficult, even if they have requested an appointment and really want to discuss some problem. If the counselee has come voluntarily, a comment such as "What would you like to talk about today?" or "Now, you wanted to talk to me?" can get things started. Very often the counselee will respond by saying, "I just don't know where to start." At such times it might be good to show understanding: "Probably a lot of things all tie in together," and then to encourage the person: "Start any place and eventually we will get the whole picture," or "Begin where it seems easiest." These statements, of course, are merely examples of a number of appropriate comments.

Occasionally a person wants to talk about some problem but is reluctant to mention it. Students may request help for a "friend," or information for a term paper they are writing on homosexuality or some similar topic. A tactful suggestion that a problem may be personal will sometimes bring denials, but often this will give the counselee the encouragement he needs to start talking.

Listen attentively Church leaders spend a lot of their time talking. This, after all, is an important part of their job, but too often it carries over into interviews as the counselor feels that he must be constantly giving wise advice or asking a lot of questions. Such an attitude greatly hinders good counseling.

When we learn to listen, the counselee has the opportunity to express his feelings, "let off steam," or "get things off his chest." In so doing, he often feels better, and at the same time gives us valuable information that we might have missed otherwise.

Watch carefully A good counselor can learn a great deal by carefully observing the counselee's speech and actions. Sometimes we see inconsistencies or gaps in a story. The person who says he is happy in his work but later talks about changing jobs, or the person who describes his family but forgets to mention his father, may be revealing something that we might ask about later.

The opening statement can also be revealing. "My mother sent me," gives a clue that the counselee may be somewhat less than enthusiastic about talking with a counselor.

There is an old saying that "actions speak louder than words," and this is true in many counseling situations. Tears or near tears, fighting, shifts in posture, or changes in breathing can all be clues that the person is dealing with important emotional issues.

At this point someone may ask, "Why do all this detective work? Why don't we just deal with the guy's problem?" This would be ideal if every counselee first had an understanding of what his real problem and, second, if every counselee were willing and able to share his problem. Very frequently, however, neither of these conditions exists.

Don't be afraid of silence When nothing is being said, most of us feel very uncomfortable; but in counseling such silence is often very meaningful. It may indicate that the counselee is struggling to control an emotion, thinking about an important issue, or debating whether to tell you more. At such times an understanding comment like "it's hard to talk sometimes isn't it?" or an encouraging remark such as "Take your time" can let the counselee know that it is all right to be silent.

Question wisely Beginning counselors often make the mistake of asking too many questions. It is best to use questions sparingly and to think before you ask. Use the following guidelines:

1 *Ask open-ended questions.*
An open-ended question is very broad and gives the counselee plenty of opportunity to respond with his opinions or further information. "How did you feel about failing?" or "What do you think now about your religious training?" or "What happened next?" are broad questions which stimulate further discussion. In contrast, "closed" questions like "Were you frustrated because you failed?" "Do you think your religious training was not relevant?" or "Is that the end of your story?" invite a one-word answer like "yes." Then the counselor feels inclined to ask another question.

2 *Avoid either-or questions.*
"Do you want to get married or stay single?" presents two alternatives. The counselee responds with his preference and the discussion stops.

3 *Try to use indirect questions.*
Direct questions are straight queries; indirect questions inquire without seeming to do so. "How does it feel to have your marriage breaking up?" is direct. "I wonder how it feels to have your marriage breaking up" is indirect. Both of these require an answer and both show the counselor's interest, but the indirect question keeps the counselee from feeling that he is being quizzed.[10]

Learn how to respond Porter has suggested that there are five commonly used counselor responses: evaluative, interpretative, supportive, probing, and understanding.[11] *Probing* responses are used when more information is needed or when the counselor wants to stimulate further discussion. With *understanding* responses, the counselor wants to convey his comprehension and empathy. By using *supportive* comments, the counselor tries to reassure or encourage the counselee. *Interpretative* responses are meant to teach the counselee or show him what is happening, while *evaluative* responses indicate what the counselor thinks about the goodness, rightness or wisdom of an action or idea. To this we might add *action* responses in which the counselor tries to encourage or stimulate the counselee to engage in some kind of action.

Although it tends to be over-used by some pastoral counselors, the *reflective* type of comment is also appropriate at times. Here the counselor tries to reflect the counselee's feelings by repeating or slightly rephrasing the counselee's statements. Such responses indicate that we understand feelings and are encouraging further conversation.

In counseling, all types of responses should be used at times, although one or two may predominate in any given interview. In addition to these verbal responses, such things as head nods, approving looks and smiles, or even periods of silence can stimulate further discussion or convey to the counselee how we are reacting.

Make use of spiritual resources Two of the greatest weaknesses of pastoral counselors are an over and under use of spiritual resources. Some Christians are of the opinion that reading the Bible or saying a prayer is all that is needed for successful counseling. Sometimes this is all that is needed, but in most cases such an approach is likely to be unsuccessful and frustrating to the counselee. It also gives the impression that Bible reading and prayer are magic charms that suddenly make everything right. At the other extreme are pastoral counselors who tend to ignore prayer and the Scriptures in their counseling, using psychological techniques almost exclusively.

Once again, no hard and fast rules can be given for the use of prayer or Bible reading. Many Christian counselors pray aloud at the beginning and/or end of an interview, and sometimes they "feel led" to pray at other times. Paul Tournier, the famous Swiss counselor, likes to have a period of "quiet communion" during which both parties silently acknowledge the presence and influence of God.[12] When it seems relevant, the counselor may also want to read a Bible passage during an interview. Narramore feels this makes more of an impression if the Bible is handed to the counselee and he is asked to read the indicated portion.[13] For this, a modern-language version may be especially helpful and, whatever the translation, it is usually wise to discuss the meaning of a passage after it is read. Christian counselees should also be encouraged to spend time daily in Bible reading, prayer, and quiet meditation. The extent to which spiritual resources will be used in counseling depends on the counselor, the counselee and the problem.

End positively It is desirable to end an interview smoothly, and, when possible, to have the counselee go away with feelings of hope and encouragement. But occasionally this is difficult and counselors are sometimes at a loss to know how a counseling session should be stopped.

If things are moving smoothly, it is wise to give the counselee a hint that the time is up. By keeping a clock on the desk or on a distant wall it is possible to keep track of the time without having to keep glancing at your watch. A statement like "Our time is just about up" gives the counselee a warning but indicates that there is still time to pick up loose ends. In the remaining minutes it may be helpful to summarize what the counselee should do next. Sometimes a word of encouragement or a short prayer is appropriate.

Occasionally counselees will raise a significant matter during these last few minutes. This may be an attempt to prolong the interview, or it may reflect the counselee's desire to raise issues at "a safe" time when it is not possible to discuss the matter further. At such times a comment such as "That would be something we could discuss next time" prevents the interview from continuing, and gives a good opener for your next session.

After the interview

When the counselee leaves, the counselor should jot down some notes and briefly evaluate the interview. This should be done immediately so that details are not forgotten. When your reactions and a summary of the session are recorded on paper, you have a convenient "memory jogger" to consult before the next interview.

The counselor must keep the interview in his confidence. Some pastors are sincerely amazed that even though their availability is well-advertised still nobody comes for counseling. Frequently these are the men who like to describe counseling cases in sermons or who let counseling details slip into other casual conversations. Even when the names and details are changed, counselees and prospective counselees often decide to go for counseling to a person who will keep quiet. At times, of course, the counselor may wish to discuss the situation with a more experienced counselor for helpful suggestions, but these confidants should be few and selected with extreme care. If a pastor's wife cannot keep quiet, for example, she cannot expect to know anything about her husband's counseling ministry.

Other considerations

Appointments At times a Christian counselor is needed immediately and without warning. When a loved one dies or a person suddenly becomes ill, the pastor must be available to offer whatever help or support he can. For most other counseling, however, it is best to set a specific prearranged appointment. This is more convenient for everyone involved. Professional counselors limit the length of an interview to fifty minutes. There is nothing sacred about this, but many experienced counselors feel that when a session is longer, less is accomplished.

Keeping records Counselors differ in the extent to which they become involved with note-taking during an interview. If he wants to take notes, the counselor might make a matter-of-fact comment at the start of the interview, such as "I'd like to jot down a few things as we talk, so I can keep the whole picture in mind." Then, during the interview he should limit his writing to brief statements which can be elaborated later. Notes taken during and after an interview should be kept in a locked cabinet. If this is not possible, it is probably best that records not be kept at all.

Psychological tests Some of these tests - measuring intelligence, interests, special abilities or personality - give results which could be helpful. The disadvantage is that the administration and interpretation of such tests are usually skilled and time-consuming tasks. However, questionnaires designed for use in pastoral counseling are especially helpful in giving background information about a counselee. Test results, like other records, should be kept confidential and locked in a safe place.

COUNSELING ETHICS

Every counselor, professional or nonprofessional, should be concerned about his ethical responsibilities and obligations. As Christians, we are responsible to God, and to the counselee and the community, for all that we do in a counseling situation. If a counselee informs us that he plans to commit murder, for example, we have an obligation to interfere to protect the counselee and his proposed victim. Many ethical decisions are not that clear-cut, however, and we must search the Scriptures and seek for the guidance of the Holy Spirit as we decide what to do in a given situation.

The following broad guidelines are basic "musts" for any pastoral counselor:

Keep confidences What is told in confidence should be kept in confidence. This means that information should not be shared without the counselee's permission, and that material from interviews generally should not be presented as sermon illustrations. The good counselor also avoids discussing one counselee and his problems with another counselee.

Recognize your limitations Apart from Jesus, no one counselor ever has the ability and training to help everyone who needs or wants help. Some people should be referred to a more experienced counselor, or to a lawyer, medical doctor, or other specialist.

Avoid physical contact Apart from a handshake, it is usually best to avoid touching a counselee. Sometimes sexual and other emotional involvement begins - at least in the counselee's mind - when physical contact is permitted.

Do not use counselees to satisfy your own desires The counselor's need for people to depend on him, for example, often influences his counseling. An understanding of one's own weak points as well as reliance on the Holy Spirit help the counselor to avoid such temptations.

Do not try to hide your Christian values The counselor's beliefs will enter everything he does, including his counseling. It is only fair to the counselee, therefore, that he have some knowledge of his counselor's Christian commitment. To do otherwise is a form of dishonesty.

Do not force or pressure the counselee to continue counseling We can encourage people to get counseling, but the person who does not want help will probably not change - regardless of the counselor.

DANGERS IN COUNSELING

In counseling, there are a number of hidden dangers. When we are aware of them, we are less likely to run into difficulties that might otherwise seriously hinder our counseling effectiveness. Some of the more common dangers in counseling include the following:

Overreliance on one-sided information All of us describe events and problems *as we see them* from our own perspective. In counseling, we usually hear only one side of an issue – the counselee's – but this may be only part of the story. In some situations, such as in marriage and family counseling, we should try to get the views of others involved.

Jumping to premature conclusions The counselor must listen attentively and avoid making early conclusions about a problem and its solutions. By trying to move too quickly, we may waste a lot of time and mental energy, since the problem which the counselee describes at first may not be the real or most pressing problem.

Over-involvement It is difficult for compassionate and sensitive people to be objective in their counseling. Too often we are tempted to shoulder the problems of other people and to get overly involved emotionally. Motives for this may be noble, but such over-involvement is emotionally and physically wearing. It interferes with our family relationships and hinders our effectiveness in dealing with non-counseling responsibilities.

Close associations with the opposite sex Just because a counselor is a Christian there is no guarantee he will never be stimulated by members of the opposite sex.

> One of the counselor's hardest tasks is to keep the counselee from becoming attached to him or her; and if the readiness

for emotional attachment is present on the counselor's side too, the counseling relationship is irreparably ruined.[14]

Techniques such as keeping the door slightly ajar as you counsel or having other people in the building are a good safeguard.

Information slips In spite of the counselor's best intentions, there is always a danger that he will inadvertently reveal some confidential information. To avoid this, we should make it a practice not to talk about other people (James 3:1-10; Peter 3:10).

A lopsided ministry Sometimes the minister or other religious worker so enjoys his counseling that he begins to neglect his other responsibilities. Counseling is an important part of the ministry, and the church leader should strive to be as effective a counselor as possible. But he must remember that, unless he is involved in a specialized counseling ministry, he also has responsibility for Bible teaching, the preparation of sermons, and other leadership tasks in the church.

2

The Counseling Procedure

Even when they have a knowledge of counseling techniques, pastoral counselors experience "deep feelings of frustration, uncertainty, and even a sense of personal uselessness when called upon for help."[1] Frequently when people pour out their problems, the church leader is so unsure about what to do that he feels incompetent and highly insecure.

How does one build confidence and overcome these feelings of frustration and insecurity? One answer appears to be "time and experience." As he counsels with a variety of people and grows in maturity, the counselor becomes more proficient and self-assured.

PHASES IN COUNSELING

It is somewhat artificial to divide a counseling relationship into steps or phases because the boundaries between such phases are vague and there is considerable overlapping. Nevertheless, for the sake of discussion we can consider counseling as having contact, introductory, problem delineation, solution, and termination phases. All these phases may take place in one interview or they may be spread over several meetings.

Making contact

Obviously we can't counsel if we never come into contact with the people who need help. In launching a counseling ministry, therefore, we must begin by letting people know of our availability. This may be done in two ways: by announcing our willingness to counsel, and by informally demonstrating our concern. Chatting over coffee or on the way home from a meeting often gives prospective counselees an opportunity to casually raise a problem issue which might later be discussed in a more formal way. If continued discussion of the problem seems wise, a comment like "Let's get together tomorrow around four o'clock so we can discuss this further," is a casual but nevertheless effective way of making an appointment.

The introductory phase

At the beginning it is very important to put the counselee at ease and to establish *rapport* – "a comfortable . . . relationship of mutual confidence between two or more persons."[2] During the introductory phase there will be a mutual "sizing up" in which both counselor and counselee look each other over and make some tentative conclusions about their relationship. If the "sizing up" leads to some mutually positive feelings, the beginnings of rapport have been established.

Early in the interview the counselee is encouraged to describe some of his symptoms and tell why he has come for counseling. The counselor should spend most of his time listening and watching. This lets him get some picture of the person, his problems and his way of looking at the world, and also permits the counselee to release some of his bottled-up emotions.

Problem delineation

As we listen to the counselee, we will begin to appreciate his problems and, hopefully, be able to see things from his point of view. The counselor might try to discover (by asking, if necessary) why the counselee has come for help, what he expects from counseling, and what he has done to solve his problems in the past. In addition, the Christian counselor may want to know something about the counselee's spiritual background. Is he a believer? Has he invited Christ to be Lord of his life? Is he rebelling against his Christian upbringing? As he talks, the counselee's statement of the problem should be accepted tentatively, but we should also be alert to the possibility that the "presented" problem* may not be the real problem.

This phase may take several counseling sessions, or it may only take a few minutes. Sometimes the counselor may feel that he doesn't fully understand why a problem has developed but if he has a clear picture of the problem itself he is still capable of helping the counselee work toward its solution.

* *Presentation problems* – in counseling situations – those problems raised in early discussions, which may prove to have little bearing on the *real* problem. Perhaps the counselee is uncertain "*how to begin,*" perhaps he needs assurance of confidentiality, perhaps he fears criticism or harsh judgment.

Working toward solutions

Young counselors often become very concerned lest they be unable to find a solution to the counselee's problem. This concern arises from the idea that counseling is like a medical relationship - the patient lists the symptoms and the doctor will provide the cure.

Counseling is not usually like this. Instead the counselee elaborates on his problem, and *both* the counselor and counselee try to work toward a solution. Often because of his objectivity, training and experience, the counselor will think of things that the counselee has never considered and many of these ideas will be discussed together by the participants. As both get greater insight into the situation, they might consider how the problem has been handled unsuccessfully in the past, and how it might be dealt with more effectively in the future. In pastoral counseling there will be a concern about the counselee's spiritual situation, and a consideration of how Christ can make a difference in troubled lives.

However, we must do more than talk about possible solutions. Each must be tried out and later evaluated by the counselee - with or without the counselor's help. If something doesn't work, we must look at the problem again and re-evaluate our past thinking.

Termination

When both participants have an understanding of the problem, have "talked it out," and hopefully have arrived at some workable solutions, there is a mutual decision to end the counseling relationship. Then the participants can discuss together how the counselee can handle his problem with a minimum of outside help. This is the real goal of the whole counseling relationship: to assist the counselee to deal more effectively on his own with the problems of life.

On paper this may sound concise and relatively easy, but it is much more difficult to apply in practice. It is helpful to remember that the counselor is not solely responsible for solving the problem but that counseling is a relationship in which at least two people are working *together* on an issue. It should also be remembered that the "phases of counseling" do not always proceed in order. Rapport is important during the entire counseling relationship, for example, and not just at the beginning.

TYPES OF COUNSELING

Supportive counseling

Church leaders, especially pastors, often find themselves giving support and encouragement in times of need. Supportive counseling is most often used with people who are having difficulty standing alone amid the problems of life. Alcoholics, for example, often need such support. Others who normally get along quite well may "fall apart" in times of crisis and need someone to lean on while they adjust to a disappointing failure, the loss of a loved one, or some other catastrophe.

In supportive counseling, the goal is not to encourage immature dependency on another person. Rather, the counselor gives temporary support and helps the person to "gain strength and perspective which will allow him to use his personality resources more effectively in coping with life situations."[3] Discourage the counselee from denying a problem exists. It is more healthy if he can be helped to face the problem realistically and attempt to understand it; express and discuss his resentments, guilt or other negative feelings; accept some responsibility for coping with the problem; explore various ways to handle the situation; recognize and accept the fact that some things cannot be changed (such as the death of a loved one); communicate with relatives, friends, and others. In all these he may be helped toward taking practical steps, however small, to handle the problem constructively.[4]

Confrontational counseling

In his dealings with people, Jesus often confronted them with their sins. He confronted the rich young ruler with his overconcern for riches (Luke 18:22), the Samaritan woman with her immorality (John 4:17-18), His disciples with their little faith (Matthew 8:26; 14:31), and the religious leaders with their sin (Matthew 12:34; John 8:44-45).

It is one thing for Jesus "who knew no sin" to be pointing out the sins of others, but it is quite another thing for Christians who have beams in their eyes to be confronting other men with their weaknesses. However, for the Christian it is clear that we must encourage people to face up to their sins. Hiding one's immoral actions only creates guilty frustration and neurotic anxiety. If we confess our sins, God will forgive (1 John 1:9), and we will obtain mercy (Proverbs 28:13). As a servant of God, the counselor must help the counselee to face his sins, to confess them, and to do something about changing himself.

Educative counseling

Most human behavior is learned behavior. We learn how to talk, think, dress, and act in social situations. When problems come into our lives we draw upon past learning to work out a solution, or we avoid the problems by using defensive mechanisms or other learned escapist techniques.

If so much behavior has been learned, it seems reasonable to assume that counseling should consist primarily of education in which the ineffective behavior is unlearned and the counselee learns more appropriate ways of acting.[5] Whether or not *all* counseling is basically relearning is another issue for debate, but there can be no doubt that *much* of the pastoral counselor's work involves education.

In educative counseling we must maintain a spirit of humility and make it our practice to look to the authoritative Word of God whenever this has a bearing on the problem. We should ask God for wisdom as we help others with their problems and we must, at times, confess that we don't know the answer but will seek to find it as we work on the problem along with the counselee.

Preventive counseling

Counseling does not exist solely for the purpose of getting people out of trouble. Sometimes its goal is to keep people from getting into trouble. Marriage counseling, for example, is usually concerned about helping partners who are having difficulty in getting along, but premarital counseling tries to anticipate problems before they arise and to help couples avoid or deal with potentially disruptive situations. The latter is preventive counseling. In it an attempt is made to anticipate problems before they arise or to deal with beginning problems before they get worse.

In our society people are not always enthusiastic about accepting unsolicited advice. This is especially true of youth who, as those most able to profit from the advice of others, are the least inclined to accept it. The counselor needs the utmost tact. He must avoid an attitude of superiority and must not convey the idea that "if you don't do this, you'll be sorry!" For example, in premarital counseling, prefer - "Have you had a chance yet to discuss how you will handle finances?" to - "Let me give you some points about handling money."

Spiritual counseling

In one sense all pastoral counseling is really spiritual counseling. As followers of Christ, we are duty-bound to make disciples of all men and to help those who are weak (Matthew 28:19-20; Romans 15:1; Galatians 6:1-2; 1 Thessalonians 5:14). Because of this, we cannot be timid in raising spiritual issues, even when the presented problem seems to be of a nonspiritual nature (such as a request for information). A question like "How are things going spiritually?" can often introduce the spiritual issue when it has not come up otherwise. In helping people find meaning and purpose in life, the religious counselor has no peer. Even Freud recognized this. "Only religion," he wrote, "is able to answer the question of the purpose of life. One can hardly go wrong in concluding that the idea of a purpose in life stands and falls with the religious system."[6] However, what appears to be a spiritual issue is often a cover for a deeper psychological problem. Hospitalized psychotics often talk about having committed the unpardonable sin, for example, but the nature of the problem is likely to be more psychological than spiritual. It is also true that many people develop psychological problems as a cover for their spiritual problems. And so, the causes of each problem may be varied and complex – but the fact that the counselee has chosen a religious counselor may indicate that there is a conscious or unconscious spiritual need.

Referral counseling

It is not an admission of failure or incompetence to refer a counselee to someone better trained to handle a problem. On arrival in a new community a pastor should begin a file of competent specialists to whom counselees could be referred by himself and by laymen involved in counseling.

There are several basic guidelines for making referrals. First, the counselor must keep the counselee's best welfare in mind. If we ask at every stage, "What is best for him?" the referral is likely to arise more smoothly. Second, the referral must be done in such a way that the counselee does not feel rejected. Frequently it takes considerable courage for a counselee to come and talk about a personal problem. The fact that he came to you indicated that, in his opinion, you are the person who can help best; so when you suggest referral, he may feel rejection and discouragement because the counselor he trusts most cannot help. To make referral easier, the counselor must do everything he can to reassure the counselee that this is the best way to deal with the problem. Third, the counselee should be part of the decision to refer. The counselor can discuss the situation with him, outline what other help is available, and indicate why it might be better to refer. Finally, the church leader should maintain a concern about the counselee and his welfare. Someone else may be doing the counseling, but the church leader is still interested.[7]

Informal counseling

Counseling doesn't always take place in the formal atmosphere of a pastor's study. On the contrary, a great deal - perhaps most - of pastoral counseling is informal. It takes place over coffee, in a hospital room, during informal home visits, or in the hallway after a meeting. Opportunities for informal counseling are many, especially if the church leader is sensitive to subtle signs of distress (such as a decline in church attendance, depression, an avoidance of people, frequent intoxication, or any other change in behavior). This informal counseling may not seem to be very important, but it has helped innumerable people. It is a way of ministering to the needy and, in so doing, we are serving the risen Christ (Matthew 25:37-40).

Group counseling

Groups have proved an effective means of pastoral counseling. By meeting with several counselees at once, the group leader makes better use of his time, and more important, provides an environment where a number of people can work together to honestly show their feelings and help each other with problems. Group counseling has greatly increased in recent years.

Christian group meetings began with the twelve disciples and were a typical characteristic of the early believers. In these church groups, which existed for the purpose of study, fellowship, communion services and prayer, the participants shared their possessions with each other, worshipped together, ate together, and spent time praising God (Acts 2:42-47). Today there is a "small-group" explosion in the church as more and more believers are meeting together to share their experiences, to confess their faults, to pray (James 5:16) and to study the Scriptures together.[8]

Group counseling in the church has been hailed as an exciting advance for pastoral counseling. This is specially true when the group is led by someone who is competent and well-trained in group-counseling methods. But there is also danger in this! In an attempt to be honest and authentic, it is easy to be vicious and inconsiderate. Some "honesty groups" are

> Harmful, and almost invariably wind up being unchristian. The object of honesty . . . is not to reveal immoral and lascivious incidents. The object is rather to begin to acknowledge to God and to each other the true nature of the personal struggles of living in the world today, so that we can begin to find freedom, healing, and forgiveness – and provide a place where others can experience these things. One does not rip off his mask (or anyone else's). Rather he becomes willing for God to remove the unnecessary part of his facade gradually by providing the security he needs to be more honest. Also a ground rule in this type of group is never to share something in such a way that it may make another person vulnerable. The highest value in the Christian life is not honesty – but *love* (1 Corinthians 13).[9]

Before suggesting group counseling, a personal interview should be held with each participant. This allows the group counselor to get some understanding of the problem and permits him to evaluate how the counselee might fit into a group. If group counseling seems advisable, a few minutes should be spent discussing with the counselee and giving him some idea of what to expect from a group.

When the group meets for the first time, the counselor may suggest some brief guidelines, such as honest sharing in love, or that group discussion be kept confidential and not reported with non-group members. Then some time should be spent in introductions, followed perhaps by a discussion of the anxiety that most people feel at the beginning of a group experience. Slowly people will begin to share their experiences and later their feelings and problems. At times they also may wish to pray together for God's guidance.

The counselor who serves as a group leader is both a participant, an observer and a catalyst. At times he expresses his own feelings, but he also tries to stimulate discussion, to occasionally summarize what is going on, and to keep the participants from wondering too far from the topic.

THE CHURCH'S COUNSELING PROGRAM

Although many people bring their problems to the church, it should always be remembered that the church is not primarily a mental health agency. Every Christian leader must ask, therefore, how the church can minister to the counseling needs of people but still carry on with its other programs of witness and work. Here are three steps in this direction:

Train pastors in counseling Most seminarians and other training institutions now offer required courses in counseling and there are frequently "pastor's courses" for men who are active in the ministry but in need of more counseling training. The professional church leader should take advantage of these educational opportunities and read broadly in the area of pastoral psychology and counseling.

Train laymen in counseling The layman is often in a crucial position for doing counseling, especially of the informal type. The pastor or professional Christian counselor can often train some of these men and women in theology, in basic psychology, and in effective counseling techniques. Such training is best restricted to more mature Christian leaders who naturally show some of the characteristics of good counselors. The person who cannot keep confidences, or the one who appears to have difficulties in relationships, should be discouraged from counseling, but encouraged to serve in some other part of the church's program.

Evaluate frequently As faithful Christian stewards, we must pause frequently to evaluate what we are doing – both as individual counselors and as a local church. After each interview, ask yourself, "What did I do that was good? What did I do that was poor? How could I have improved the counseling?" At a more general level, church leaders can periodically ask themselves if they are meeting the needs of the people, helping them with their problems, and assisting them in their spiritual growth.

II

Situations in Counseling

3

Premarital, Marital and Family Counseling

When God created the heavens and the earth, He ordained that human beings should be of two sexes, male and female (Genesis 1:27). Adam and Eve became the first married couple and soon they began raising children. Beginning with their example, the importance of marriage and the family is stressed time and time again throughout the pages of Scripture. The family is mentioned in all sixty-six books of the Bible; guidelines for successful family living appear frequently (see especially Ephesians 5:22-6:4); and there are numerous examples of family relationships. The Bible describes the family backgrounds of great leaders such as Abraham, Isaac, Jacob, Joseph, Moses, Samuel, David, John the Baptist, and a host of others, including Jesus Himself. Although He never married, Jesus clearly approved of marriage (John 2:1-11) and later He commented on the ideal of Christian marriage as a lifelong union in which two people become one (Mark 10:5-9).

In a survey conducted several years ago it was found that 50 percent of all people who came to a pastor for counseling did so because of marriage or family problems.[1]

More recently in surveys of church youth it was found that young people listed dating and marriage as the topics for which, more than any other, they wanted help from the church.[2] It is hardly surprising, then, that Clinebell, after reviewing the whole issue of marriage and family counseling, concluded that proficiency in this area should be the church leader's "most indispensable counseling skill."[3]

PREMARITAL COUNSELING

The time to begin work on marriage and family problems is before they ever arise. Ideally, preparation for marriage begins when one is a small child. If the parents have a good marriage, the children learn attitudes and ways of behaving which enable them in turn to also have happy marriages.[4]

Regardless of one's home background, however, the decision to marry is of major importance and many couples approach their wedding day with feelings of both expectant enthusiasm and fearful hesitation. By helping people at this critical time in their lives, the church leader is often able to make a significant contribution to the future success of these marriages.

Gospels of premarital counseling

Premarital counseling seeks to help individuals, couples, and groups of couples to prepare for and build happy and successful marriages. Just as preventive medicine attempts to prevent disease and point people toward health, so premarital guidance seeks to anticipate difficulties in marriage and family living and to help people build healthy, satisfying marriage relationships.[5] In counseling with people prior to marriage, at least five goals are of special importance.[6]

To assess readiness for marriage While there is no concise formula by which to determine if a person is ready for marriage, here are some broad indicators which the counselor should bear in mind:

1 *The reasons for marriage*
An engaged couple may present any number of sound reasons for getting married, including love, an awareness of God's leading, or a desire for companionship and sexual fulfillment. Sometimes, however, the stated reasons are such that a marriage would be unwise. It is especially difficult for a husband and wife to build a good relationship if they marry primarily as a response to social pressure, to show revenge against a parent or former partner, to avoid the stigma of being an "old maid," to get away from an unhappy home, to satisfy sexual infatuations, or because the girl is pregnant.

2 *The degree of background similarity*
A marriage is more likely to be successful when a couple have similar interests and values, comes from the same socioeconomic class and similar family backgrounds, are of the same race, have a similar amount of education, and are of the same religious faith.[7]

3 *Age*
A number of research studies have shown that teenage marriages are not very stable and end in divorce much more often than do marriage between couples who are

older.[8] These marriages are plagued with problems from the beginning and the participants are often not mature enough to handle the stress. Maturity does not always come automatically with age, but the older one gets, the greater the likelihood that one can establish and maintain personal relationships and effectively meet the problems of life.[9]

4 *In addition to age in terms of years, there is also the issue of age differences*

Difficulties are more likely if the couple is ten or more years apart. In such cases there are often dissimilarities in interests and physical vigor, a difficulty in finding mutual friends, and a tendency for the older person to act as a parent rather than as a spouse.[10]

5 *Courtship*

The period of courtship and engagement is an important predictor of later marital success. The couple who have known each other for a short time, or whose courtship has been stormy and characterized by frequent conflict are not ready for marriage.[11]

6 *Attitudes towards marriage*

If a person is afraid of or repulsed by thoughts of sexual intercourse, if there is a strong fear of marriage, if there is disagreement about whether or not to have children, if the prospective bride and groom have different views of the roles that each will assume in marriage, or if there are differing plans and expectations for the future, then it would surely be wise to postpone the wedding until these attitudes can be "talked through," – perhaps with a counselor's help.

7 *External circumstances*
Sometimes there are circumstances in life which put added strain on a young marriage. These include demands imposed by further schooling, existence of large debts, pressures of limited finances, or parental opposition.[12]

8 *Spiritual maturity*
Regardless of the above considerations, an individual is not ready for Christian marriage if he is an unbeliever, if he wants to marry a non-Christian, or if he is not completely yielded to the lordship of Jesus Christ. When we become believers we give ourselves to Christ, we become His children, and seek to do His will. If we marry someone who has a different commitment, either the marriage will suffer or our Christian service will be less effective. It is important, therefore, that the believer seek another of like precious faith and that they walk together as one, serving Christ together. This mutual spiritual concern is no guarantee of automatic marital success (Christian and non-Christians alike can have problems and must work at marriage), but there are sure to be difficulties if one seeks to be a committed believer while "unequally yoked" with one who is spiritually dead (2 Corinthians 6:14).

To anticipate potential stress Closely associated with determining a person's readiness for marriage is the task of identifying potential areas of stress. When two people of the opposite sex with different family backgrounds and varied past experiences begin to share life together, there are sure to be some adjustment problems. If these can be anticipated before marriage, the adjustment is likely to be much easier.

Issues which put stress on a marriage will differ from one couple to another, but some problems are especially common. In one widely reported study of several hundred married people, for example, it was found that the most difficult areas of marital adjustment were sexual adjustment, the handling of finances, the choice of social and recreational activities, problems of getting along with in-laws, differences in religious values or beliefs, and conflicts over the choice of friends - in that order.[13] Long before the wedding day, a prospective bride and groom should be alerted to these issues and encouraged to discuss them openly, honestly and at length. The attitudes and expectations that each has about these problem areas should be aired, with attempts made to resolve conflicts. It is not of great importance whether the issues are discussed by the couple alone, with other engaged persons in a group, or in the presence of a counselor. What is important is that the issues get discussed in depth, and that accurate factual knowledge be available for those who need it.

If the counselor is to help couples anticipate the stresses of marriage, he would be wise to also encourage them to give careful thought to the honeymoon.

The honeymoon is a transition stage between single and married life. It is an opportunity for the newly married couple to relax with each other and to start - psychologically and physically - to get used to their new status. However, even when a honeymoon is carefully planned and eagerly anticipated, there is always a degree of awkwardness. Inhibitions take time to overcome and it is probable that, in spite of the joys of the honeymoon, sexual adjustments during those first few days are at the poorest level that they will ever be.[14]

It cannot be emphasized too strongly that most of the problems before and during marriage can be adequately met if a couple learns to communicate. Certainly it takes effort to listen carefully, to try to understand accurately, and to express oneself honestly in an attitude of love and mutual respect. The end result, however, is a smoother marital relationship, and this makes the effort worthwhile. Communication of one's attitudes, feelings, frustrations and uncertainties is as important as the communication of love and respect, but such communication does not start on the honeymoon. It begins long before marriage, and the premarital counselor should do everything in his power to encourage and guide in the development of communication ability.

To guide self-evaluation In any interpersonal situation – including marriage – relationships are likely to be smoother if the participants are able to take an honest look at themselves. Jesus may have had this in mind when he told His followers to look at the planks in their own eyes before picking out the specks in others (Matthew 7:3-5). The problem with this is that self-appraisal is painful and likely to make us feel uncomfortable. Nobody likes to face up to his own faults; it's much easier to criticize someone else. When disagreements arise during the engagement period and later in marriage, the natural tendency is to self-righteously blame the other for most if not all of the problems, and then to push for one's own way. It never occurs to some people that at least part of the blame might be theirs.

To consider biblical views of marriage Shortly after man was created, God made woman. "It is not good that the man should be alone," the Creator decreed, so He instituted marriage and declared that a man should "cleave unto his wife; and they should be one flesh" (Genesis 2:18, 24).

With the help of the pastoral counselor, the couple should carefully discuss these divine ideals, especially as they are outlined in Ephesians 5:21-6:4, Colossians 3:16-21, 1 Corinthians 7, and 1 Peter 3:1-7. Since the relationship of the husband and wife is modeled after the bond that Christ has with his church, the latter should also be fully understood. Such an understanding makes it easier for many Christians to accept and appreciate such passages as those which instruct the wife to be in subjection to her husband. In these days of Women's Liberation, the biblical view is very unpopular and even some Christians prefer to eliminate "obey" from the wedding ceremony. But the husband's being "head of the wife" does not imply aggressive and cruel domination. Instead, it means a sacrificial and giving love like that described in 1 Corinthians 13. The wife, in turn, responds not as a resentful and brutalized slave, but rather in cheerful submission to the one who is as concerned about her and her happiness as he is about himself.[15]

To plan the wedding In our culture, planning a wedding is a major undertaking which involves decisions about flowers, attendants, dresses, photographers, the reception, the cake, the guest list and, for many, how all of this can be paid for. As a couple approaches the wedding day, the premarital counselor has three major responsibilities. *First,* he can encourage the participants to 'take it easy' in their planning.

Second, the counselor must insure that the couple meet the legal requirements for marriage. This usually involves getting a license and in some countries having a blood test or other physical examination.

Third, the counselor - in this case the pastor - can go over the service in detail prior to the wedding. For most people their marriage ceremony is a climax to weeks of planning, but frequently the main participants are too tired or too emotionally "keyed up" to remember much of what is being said. It is important, therefore, that the service be discussed in detail beforehand in order that the meaning of the pastor's statements be understood, and that the spiritual aspects of the service be considered. If the couple are Christians they should realize that the wedding can be an important witness of their mutual commitment to Christ. For many this realization has an influence on the music that is selected and on other details of the service.

Techniques of premarital counseling

Whenever a church leader has the opportunity of speaking to a youth group about Christian marriage, dating or sex, he is involved in a form of premarital counseling. Most teenagers and single adults are vitally interested in their relationships with the opposite sex. As they date, these young people are forming attitudes about the other sex and learning how to relate to each other.

A second opportunity for premarital counseling comes with the establishing of discussion groups or classes for engaged couples. Such groups should not be too large (four or five couples is ideal) and should be limited to couples who have already decided to get married. At their first meeting, the participants might each give a thumbnail sketch of themselves and then discuss how the groups will proceed. Ideally, the format and subject matter should be flexible although it is wise to have at least some ground rules. For example, each couple should agree to come for as many meetings as possible.

While discussion among the participants should be open and honest, the subject matter of the sessions might be kept confidential from those outside of the group. On a chalkboard or notepad, the group leader should jot down issues that the couples propose for discussion, and he may add a few suggestions of his own. The nature of communication, the meaning of love, the management of finances, the use of time, the question of in-laws, the importance of the honeymoon, the issues of sex and contraceptives, the control of sexual urges before marriage, the problems of pregnancy and childbirth, the ways of handling disagreements, the existence of doubts about marriage, the role of religion in the home, and the details of the biblical view of marriage, are among the topics that should be considered.

At the completion of a group counseling series, it is good to get suggestions from the participants concerning ways for improving future counseling. Often this feedback can be especially helpful if the group gets together several months after the couples have been married. Such an "alumni gathering" is a good opportunity for the newly married to discuss issues that they are now facing as husband and wife.

In their premarital sessions some counselors follow a prearranged formula - a session on rapport-building and discussion of the biblical view of marriage; a session on roles, responsibilities, personality differences, and potential problems in marriage; and a session discussing details of the ceremony. While such a guideline is acceptable and often very helpful, it should not be followed too rigidly. At times it is appropriate to loan a book with the suggestion that it be circulated and read prior to the next session.[16]

SPECIAL PROBLEMS IN PREMARITAL COUNSELING

Parental disapproval of the marriage A pastor who knows all of the participants is in a tight spot in this situation. All parties may have stated good reasons for their opinions, so the counselor becomes a mediator, trying to bring about a reconciliation. It should be recognized, however, that this is one of those situations in which both sides might try to distort the counselor's words and try to "get him on our side." At times it may be appropriate to call all of the participants together and to clarify your own role in the situation.

Premarital pregnancy This situation is frequently very stressful for all involved. When he learns of the situation, the counselor should encourage the couple to inform their parents, if this has not already been done, and to get proper medical attention. Feelings of shame, guilt and disappointment often must be dealt with over a long period of time, and the couple (and their parents) should be counseled as they decide what is their next course of action. Often a local physician can give helpful information on community agencies that minister specifically to unwed mothers.

Mixed marriages In the minds of many people, "mixed marriage" refers only to a union between persons of different races, but the term can be more broadly applied. When people of different religious, socioeconomic, educational, or age groups decide to marry, their relationship can also be described as "mixed." While many of these marriages succeed, an exceptionally large number develop serious problems. Differences in family background can lead to disagreements over values, interests and routine ways of living. Add to this the ostracisms and disapproval from family and community residents, and the problems become especially difficult. If a couple are both committed Christians there is no scriptural reason why the color of their skin or the size of their bank account should prevent their getting married. In counseling with such couples, however, the church leader should make sure that they are fully aware of the difficulties involved, and he should assure them of his continued availability for counsel after the wedding.

Mental illness Should severely disturbed people be permitted to marry? Sometimes this can be good therapy, but since a marriage can be no more stable than the individual involved, the prospects for marital harmony in such cases are not very good.

Severe doubts Marriage is a lifelong commitment and because of its importance some couples approach it with real insecurity. It is common for couples to have periods of uncertainty as they approach their wedding day, and in such cases the feelings are best discussed openly and examined in the light of the present reality. Usually it is wise to pray about these feelings, realizing that God leads in every aspect of life, including marriage.

Anxiety is a mild form of discomfort and uncertainty that is experienced almost universally. The counselor can reassure distressed couples and help them to accept their feelings.

MARITAL COUNSELING

Healthy marriage has been described by Clinebell as "at once the most demanding and the most potentially rewarding" of all human relationships.[17] As husband and wife, two adults merge their separate lives into an intimate and complex union which the Bible describes as good and honorable (Proverbs 18:22; Hebrews 13:4).

Marriages, however, are not always smooth. Often there are disagreements, distrust and misunderstanding before the two parties begin to function as a unit. The merger of two people in marriage can be likened to the coming together of two great rivers. For many miles the water share the same riverbed, but only slowly is there mixing so that the two become one.

The need for marriage counseling

As you read these words, hundreds of thousands of marriages are sick and dying. Couples who went to the altar with high hopes and eager expectations have seen their marriages degenerate into tired friendship or a long drawn-out war. The reasons for this marital disharmony are both numerous and complex, but some of the more common include the following:

Lack of communication Marriage counselors consistently report that couples who aren't getting along are often unable to communicate.[18] Sometimes there is open quarreling, sometimes sullen silence, but always there is inability to honestly share feelings and ideas about significant issues. By patiently watching a couple as they interact, the counselor can often see where communication is breaking down; but to improve interaction is a difficult assignment, especially when the couple doesn't particularly want to improve their communication.

Immaturity Very often couples begin marriage with unrealistically high expectations, only to be disappointed and disenchanted when the relationship does not turn out as they had hoped. This realization can give cause for working harder at the marriage and making it a mutually satisfying experience.

For many couples, however, the disenchantment does not lead to increased efforts; instead, it encourages immature behavior that puts further strain on the marriage. Unreasonable demands, lack of consideration for the spouse's feelings, blaming the other for one's own faults, impulsive behavior, irresponsibility, intemperance, increased rigidity in one's attitudes, and an overdependency on the parents are all indications of immaturity.[19] People don't mature in a day and, even with the understanding guidance of a counselor, a marriage built on immaturity will have a long slow road to improvement.

According to the Bible, marriage is a lifelong institution, but many people today fail to accept this view. They see marriage as an arrangement of convenience which lasts "for the foreseeable future" and to be terminated at will by either or both of the parties involved. Even among married couples there may be many who feel no responsibility to remain faithful to their spouse.

Ask any couple why they plan to get married and the most common response is: "Because we are in love." If they later decide to get a divorce, one of the stated reasons is likely to be: "We don't love each other anymore." The Scriptures instruct husbands to love their wives (Ephesians 5:25) and wives to love their husbands (Titus 2:4) but what does this mean? Popular ballads, poems and movies glorify love but the term is used so broadly that it is almost meaningless.

In regard to the marital relationship, the Bible gives two examples of what love should be like: First, husbands should love their wives as Christ loved the church

(Ephesians 5:25-27). The love of Christ is unselfish, and without strings attached. As described in 1 Corinthians 13, Christian love is patient, kind, and free of jealousy, envy, boasting, pride, grudges, rudeness or self-glorification. It is a giving relationship which involves loyalty and concern for the object of one's love. This kind of love cannot be "turned on" at will, nor is it something we "fall into or out of." Love is a growing relationship which, for Christians, is an outward expression of the love of Christ in a life. Marital love is also to be similar to self-love. Men should love their wives, the Scriptures say, as they love themselves (Ephesians 5:28-33). This can hardly be consistent with the casual way in which some people view the marriage bond.

Unhealthy "need fulfillment" In any successful marriage, the participants will have certain needs fulfilled. The need for love, security, respect, acceptance, safety, and sexual fulfillment in marriage, for example, is so important, that one counselor has defined a happy marriage as "one in which there is a relatively high degree of mutual need and satisfaction," and an unhappy marriage as one with much 'need frustration.'[20] Sometimes marriages experience difficulty because one or both of the partners have needs that are not being met. In such cases, communication of the lack of fulfillment is important, and the partners can work – perhaps with the help of a counselor – to make the relationship more mutually need-satisfying.

The goals of marital counseling

In his contacts with married couples, the church leader can help in two important ways: he can guide in the building and improving of a marriage, and he can counsel with those who are having marital conflicts. In both cases, the counselor is attempting to help the partners improve their relationship with each other and with God.

These two broad goals can be subdivided into more specific aims. During the course of his counseling, the counselor should try to:

- Reopen lines of communication between the couple and to encourage the expression of feelings.
- Encourage understanding of each person's own attitudes, goals, needs and views of marriage as well as those of one's spouse.
- Help couples accept each other and stop trying to reform and transform each other.
- Interrupt the vicious cycle of mutual retaliation.
- Help the couple work together at translating their new understanding and acceptance into appropriate action so that the relationship is improved.
- Be less demanding and more responsible in relating to each other.
- Encourage commitment to Christ and a familiarity with the biblical guidelines for marital stability.

Counseling the newly married

Even when there has been good premarital counseling, the first months and years of married life can be very demanding. During this time the young husband and wife are learning to adjust to each other and to their married status. Unanticipated conflicts, irritations, and communication breakdowns may frustrate the couple who, at least in the beginning, may have been expecting consistent marital bliss. It may be discovered that, despite the careful planning before the wedding, it is not always easy to manage the money, get along smoothly with two sets of parents, or achieve a mutually satisfying sexual adjustment.[21]

Church leaders who recognize the value of premarital guidance sometimes fail to appreciate the importance of counseling after the honeymoon. If a couple can be guided during the early stages of married life, however, the marriage can be strengthened, and subsequent problems in the home can be avoided. But how does a church leader get started in counseling with newlyweds? Rarely does the couple come for counseling on their own, and they may be tired of hearing advice from well-meaning older people who have been married for a long time.

The value of counseling for the newly married should be stressed during the period of premarital counseling and perhaps at that time an appointment can be set up for sometime after the wedding. A pastoral call or two in the couple's new home gives the church leader a chance to visit the newlyweds and to ask, "How are things going now that you are married?" A Sunday school class for the newly married could provide opportunity for consideration of problem areas, or it might be helpful to establish an evening discussions group which would be attended by young couples during their first year of marriage. These get-togethers could each last for a couple of hours and could focus on issues which the group members identified as being important.[22]

Joint and individual interviews

Living together in the intimacies of marriage often leads to problems for which a couple needs help. When such marital difficulties arise, it is best for both husband and wife to participate in the counseling, although there can be value in seeing only one spouse if the other absolutely refuses to cooperate or has no desire to continue the marriage.

When a couple is seen together, the counselor has an excellent chance to observe their relationship and to see how they communicate. If both sincerely want to get along better, there can be mutual discussion of the misunderstandings, disagreements, personality characteristics, and insensitivities that are undermining the marriage. By seeing the husband and wife separately it is possible for the counselor to get a more accurate idea of what each is like and to see how each views the marriage with its problems. Because there is value in both joint and individual interviews, it is usually best to use a combination of both.

As he works with the couple, the counselor must show concern, understanding, impartiality, and a willingness to listen. This does not mean that he just nods his head and says nothing. At times the counselor must ask for information, express his understanding, point out inconsistencies, answer questions, make reference to relevant biblical principles, give counsel, and confront the counselees with some of the ways in which they are contributing to the problem.

Special areas of marital stress

While no two problem marriages have exactly the same weaknesses, the counselor encounters some issues time and time again.

Role conflicts When a couple gets married they each have expectations of what a husband and a wife are supposed to do in the marriage. These expectations arise largely from observations of how one's own parents function in their relationships. Conflicts arise almost invariably if the wife and husband think differently about whether married women should work, whether a working woman's money is hers to keep, or whether a couple should visit his parents every Christmas.

Money The love of money, according to the Scriptures, is a root of all evil (1 Timothy 6:10). Lack of money and disagreements about its use, according to several research reports, are the most common issues of conflict between husbands and wives.[23] Careful planning can prevent or at least reduce many of the financial problems of marriage. When couples have different ideas on how to spend money, the use of a wife's income, or the value of installment purchases, there must be more discussion and compromise.

In-laws When a man marries, he leaves his father and mother and cleaves to his wife (Matthew 19:5). Presumably the wife makes a similar break from her parents when she submits herself to her husband (Ephesians 5:22). In practice, of course, this transition is not nearly so precise. Instead, we talk about "marrying into a family," and as everyone knows, when a person takes a spouse, he or she also collects a whole new group of relatives. In marital counseling the attitudes of in-laws and attitudes toward in-laws should be discussed. These in-law problems sometimes are the major cause of disagreement, while at other times they lurk in the background, indirectly influencing other problems.[24] Sometimes it is necessary to accept the inevitability of a difficult in-law situation and to live with it as peacefully as we can (Romans 12:18).

Sex Sexual intercourse should be the highest expression of love between a man and a woman. Here two people cleave as "one flesh" wholly committed to each other in physical and psychological union.

For many couples this is a reality, but for others it is a fictional idea. Frigidity, impotency, inability to experience orgasm at the same time, infidelity, disagreements over the use of contraceptives, differences in sexual desires, insensitivity to each other's feelings, and a number of other problems may prevent real sexual fulfillment in a marriage. It should be emphasized that sex often gets blamed as a cause for marital difficulties when really it is a symptom of some other problem. Certainly there is no one-to-one relationship between marital instability and sexual problems, but more often than not, prolonged sexual problems reflect other kinds of difficulties between the husband and wife. When a couple is really working at their relationship and making progress in getting along, their sexual problems can be solved. Consultation with a physician, discussion with a more experienced married couple, reading a book on sex, and freely discussing feelings and frustrations with each other, all are ways in which a couple can improve the sex act if they both want a change for the better.

Pregnancy and childbirth A couple may experience mixed feelings when they learn that the wife is pregnant for the first time. There is often excitement at the prospect of parenthood, accompanied by a realization that one's style of life will soon change. If the couple have been active in doing things together, if the wife has had a good job, or if children were not wanted at this time, the early months of pregnancy can be especially difficult. The wife's physical condition may have a psychological influence so that she has periods of discouragement and weeping. All of this can put a strain on a marriage - especially an unstable one - but communication of feelings between the couple, and a willingness to understand each other can make pregnancy and the beginning of parenthood a rewarding experience.

Spiritual conflicts Research studies show that families who pray and worship together do, indeed, stay together and have a much lower separation or divorce rate than nonreligious families. But religion contributes to marital stability only insofar as it is shared by both husband and wife.[25] There are likely to be conflicts, for example, if one is deeply religious or committed to the lordship of Christ while the other is a nonbeliever or less committed. The Apostle Paul advised such couples to stay together (1 Corinthians 7:12-13) but it is to be expected that in such situations there will be differences in values, preferences for leisure activities, standards for raising children, amount of participation in church services, and interest in other religious activities.

The problem of divorce Legally there can be numerous grounds for divorce, with the laws differing from place to place. In contrast, the Bible has a more stringent set of requirements and appears to give only two grounds for divorce for the Christian: desertion by an unbeliever (1 Corinthians 7:15) and adultery (Matthew 5:32; 19:9; Luke 16:18).

While the counselor will want to do everything in his power to heal broken marriages, he must realize that at times separation or divorce is unavoidable and may be the best solution for all involved. When this happens there are likely to be considerable adjustment problems. There are often feelings of loneliness, hostility, insecurity, guilt, rejection, and loss of self-esteem. There are difficulties adjusting to the role of "divorced person" and the welfare of the children who will be from a broken home should be a major concern.

FAMILY COUNSELING

Counselors traditionally worked with individual family members. However, over the years, it became more and more apparent that something more was needed, because the value of individual counseling was often undermined when the counselee went back into the turmoil of a family in conflict. To meet this problem, some counselors began to work with the family as a group.[26] In counseling, the family members (of school age and above) meet together to discuss their mutual problems, to increase mutual understanding, and to learn how to improve communication.

The church leader may find himself involved in a simple form of family counseling whenever he makes a pastoral call. In more formal counseling the family might come to the church to meet together with the counselor. In this situation it is sometimes good to talk briefly with the parents alone, and briefly with the children alone, but most of the time should be spent with the whole family meeting together.[27] Each family member should be given the opportunity to talk about the family problems from his perspective. At first this is likely to be threatening to the participants, but as the counselor encourages openness and is himself a model of good communication, the discussion becomes freer. As with all pastoral counseling, the group leader may suggest that the family should consider one or two relevant Bible passages, and there is value in encouraging prayer together. Thus, family counseling becomes a special form of group counseling.

4

Vocational Counseling

Choosing a vocation is one of man's most significant and far-reaching decisions. Our choice of occupation determines how we will spend at least one-third of our waking hours, for this is the minimum amount of time that most people spend at work during their adult lives. Our work determines our income and this, in turn, affects one's standard of living and place of residence. The kind of work that we do and the success of our careers have an influence on the type of people we have for friends, on our status in the community and on the kind of relationships we have with our families.

The selection of an occupation has added importance for the Christian. When we acknowledge that Christ is Lord, we must turn over our whole lives - including our working lives - to His control. It becomes crucial, then, that our choice of an occupation be in accordance with divine will, and that our daily work be done diligently "as unto Christ" (Ephesians 6:5-6).

In view of the social, psychological and theological importance of work, the choice of a vocation should be made with great care and deliberation. Too often, however, the decision is made in a haphazard and hurried fashion. Parents, teachers, friends, and others in our society expect occupational decisions to be made early. Thus, at a time when they are inexperienced, idealistic, and struggling with the problems of adolescence, young people have the added responsibility of choosing from an almost unlimited number of career possibilities. Is it surprising then that so many end up dissatisfied and frustrated with their jobs?

Whenever one person talks with another about a career choice, vocational counseling is, to some extent, taking place. Whether the counseling is of this informal nature or more professional in character, it involves three basic aspects: being familiar with the world of work, knowing the counselee, and guiding in the making of decisions.

Knowing the world of work

What would you really like to accomplish in your life work? If you ask this question, people usually give one or more of the following answers: "to help people," "to get personal success in terms of money or fame," or "to express myself in some way" (as in writing or art.)[1] To achieve goals such as these, a lot of people apparently think that they must enter a profession. This is highly unrealistic and for many will lead to severe disappointment.

This kind of disappointment can be prevented if the counselor knows something about the world of work and the requirements for various occupations. But this is not an easy task. Literally thousands of job opportunities are available, and even the professional guidance counselor cannot keep fully abreast of all developments in the field. How, then, can the pastor, Sunday School teacher, or other church leader help the occupation seeker?

The answer is twofold: show him where to get information, and suggest the questions that he should ask about different jobs.

Type of information When one has located the depository of information, what sort of things does he look for as he tries to find out about jobs? This will vary from situation to situation. Some occupations are rare or obscure and we need to ferret out information. Other fields of work are well known and the counselee may only want to uncover one or two pertinent facts.

Knowing the counselee

There are many reasons why people choose to enter a specific occupation. The opinions of parents are very important - especially with younger people - but in addition there are the influence of friends or teachers, the interest that comes from hobbies and extracurricular activities, the glamour and prestige that are associated with different occupations (being a surgeon sounds much more attractive than being a used-car salesman), the information that describes various careers, and the student's evaluation of his own abilities and potentialities.

General ability In vocational counseling we must try to help the counselee set his aspirations in accordance with his ability. Usually this will involve slowing down someone whose goals are unrealistically high, but occasionally we must encourage capable people who have set their sights too low. The student's grades are often a good indication of his ability and of his potential for performance in later schooling.

Specific abilities Most of us have special abilities in at least one or two areas and these should be considered in vocational planning. Some people, for example, are mechanically inclined - they can fix anything. Others have unusual musical ability or a special way of getting along with people. Equally important are a person's noticeable weaknesses. A person who can't throw a ball obviously would be ill-advised if we encouraged a career in baseball.

Personality traits People with equal intellectual ability are not equally suited for the same occupations. Some are shy and withdrawn; others are outgoing. Some like a lot of change; others prefer life to be more orderly and routine. Some are cheerful, impulsive, active or critical, while others might be less cheerful, prone to plan carefully, and more lethargic and accepting. Personality differences such as these are very important in vocational choice and adjustment. The person who wants to be a missionary had better be flexible, accepting and able to get along with people, for example, or he is heading for trouble.

Interests Our likes and dislikes are also important in career choice. While tests give a good summary of such interests, it can also be helpful to reflect on our preferences and jot these down on a piece of paper. As a start, we might ask how we spend our spare time and money. This is an excellent barometer of one's values and gives a good clue to one's interests. It should be emphasized that the counselee should try to identify his own real interests and not simply reflect on the suggestions and aspirations of his parents or teachers.

Spiritual state The person deeply committed to Christ and wanting to serve Him in all aspects of life will approach vocational counseling with different aspirations than will the non-Christian or the half-hearted believer. The Christian counselor would certainly want to ascertain the counselee's spiritual state therefore, and at some time discuss the believer's responsibility to spend his life in service to Christ and the place of His choosing.

Guiding in the decision process

It would be convenient if the counselor could analyze the world of work, appraise the counselee's characteristics, and then announce the one perfect occupation. Such a goal is, of course, impossible.

The work of the counselor is to help the counselee acquire the needed information and to guide as he uses this to make his vocational decision. In the words of one writer,

> . . . We need to help young people learn how to make decisions which are, on the one hand, appropriate for them, and on the other hand, realistic and flexible. This means that they need to know what alternative courses of action are open to them; what are the consequences and risks of choosing each of them; and how these factors relate to their own system of values. They need to become aware that the ultimate responsibility for making choices rests with them, but that we stand ready to help them in the decision-making process. . . . We need to (and indeed must) "motivate" adolescents to make the choices, educationally and vocationally, which are feasible for them at their stage of development.[2]

SPECIAL ISSUES IN VOCATIONAL COUNSELING

The unemployed

The church is not an employment agency, but at times the pastor or other church members encounter someone who is out of work and in need of guidance in finding a job. In ministering to such people our first task is to express a sincere concern. Since it is often frustrating and discouraging to be unemployed, the church leader performs a real service by being a sympathetic listener, by reminding the counselee of God's care and concern, and by praying with the job seeker. This is not to imply that a short sermon and a prayer provide the solution to the problem and relieve the counselor of any further responsibility. The book of James warns against such a simplistic approach to the needy (James 2:14-17). However, if the unemployed person and his friend in the church consider the situation *together* and can pray together, this can be a significant step in the right direction.

Depending somewhat on the length of time that one has been unemployed, it might be helpful if the church could provide clothing, food, or other tangible help. Accepting help is often embarrassing and a threat to one's self-esteem. Because of this the church leader should be careful to insure that the gift is given in a way that is minimally embarrassing.

The dissatisfied

The child does not have to make realistic work choices but can move ahead on the assumption that when he grows up he can "be anything" he wants. The ages between about fifteen and twenty-five are labeled the *exploratory stage.* Here the person is trying to "find himself," to develop his values, and to make realistic occupational plans. He will probably select - and discard - a number of occupations before settling on one area of work. During this stage he must learn how to find a job and how to cope with the problems of adjusting to the requirements of work. This is followed by the *establishment stage* during which the worker establishes a family, a home, and a place in the community. There may be mobility during this stage, but there is less floundering. The person has found a place in the world of work and is now attempting to establish himself.

During the *maintenance stage* the individual seeks to "hold his own." Having made a place in the vocational world, he now seeks to continue his level of efficiency until the time of retirement. Although there are exceptions, most people in this period of life make no attempt to be boldy creative or to try something new. If a person has reached his life goals, this can be a time of real satisfaction. It can also be a time of frustration for the individual who didn't achieve as he had hoped and who realizes that he will be forced to lower his aspirations.

When he reaches the age of retirement, the person enters the *stage of decline.* This involves a tapering off in one's vocational activities and an adjustment to retirement.

In any of these last three stages, people may be dissatisfied with their careers. During the exploratory stage there will be floundering and frustration, but there is also hope. Eventually, the young person believes, he will find a position which is satisfying and fulfilling. As they move into the establishment and maintenance stages, however, many people are forced to face hard reality. Bischof says these adult years are "a time of truth" when the dreams and aspirations of the twenties, thirties, and early forties must give way to the reality of the present.[3] People discover that they are not succeeding as they had hoped and that they will not advance much beyond their present position. Many feel "locked in" to a dissatisfying job situation with no alternative but to wait it out until retirement.

The church leader can help the dissatisfied worker in several ways. Once again, he can express concern and be a sympathetic listener, but as he considers the situation with the counselee, it might also be wise to discuss some practical alternatives. There are at least six of these, according to Dickerson.[4]

1 **Start a new occupation.** Although many men do succeed in changing jobs in middle age, this is not easy. The job change may involve a lowering of salary, loss of seniority, necessity for retraining – and all these put extra pressure on a father supporting a wife and family. The worker who is determined to change his occupation should be alerted to the problems.

2 **Change employers.** In some occupations this is quite common and acceptable. The individual stays in the same occupation, so his experience counts, but he moves to another employer. Pastors do this frequently and so do college professors – often with an accompanying advance in salary.

3 **Change jobs within the same company.** This permits a man to retain his seniority and salary but to find working conditions or associates which are more to his liking. In some professional situations it is possible to alter one's

duties in order to re-define the job in accordance with one's preferences. Ministers, for example, might be able to emphasize some special part of their ministry - such as sermon preparation or counseling - and leave some of their remaining duties to others.

4 **Stay in the present job.** At times this may be the most feasible alternative - to stay with the problem job and to get satisfaction elsewhere. For the layman, the church is one place where there can be opportunities for rewarding and meaningful service.

5 **Change oneself.** Might it be that the problem is not so much with the work as it is with the worker? Perhaps a critical attitude, an unwillingness to cooperate, a festering resentment, an inability to accept authority, or a severe disappointment with one's job may make the situation seem worse than it really is.

6 **Change one's attitude toward work.** Sometimes Christians have the idea that unless they are in a full-time church-related occupation they are not really serving God. In certain circles, the missionary is considered to be most in God's will, followed in turn by the pastor, other full-time workers and then "those who have compromised with the world." The Bible gives no support to this thinking. Indeed, while many occupations are mentioned in Scripture, there is never a suggestion that one is better than another.[5] As Christians we must diligently serve Christ in everything that we do, including work. In our secular jobs we should serve our employers as faithfully as if we were working directly for Christ (Ephesians 6:5-8). The dignity of work well done is perhaps a value which is

fading from our society. We must remember, however, that a Christian is a witness wherever he goes.

The senior citizen

In our complex, changing technological society, with its adulation of youth, there is little place for the person who is in the stage of decline.

Coping with retirement In spite of popular notions about the "golden years," few people approach retirement enthusiastically.[6] While the prospect of freedom from work is attractive, many people fear that they will lose status, self-respect, and the companionship of co-workers when they retire. The end of one's working career almost always means a reduction of income and a corresponding decline in one's standard of living.

Finding new work There is nothing about age sixty or sixty-five that makes one old. Many people are both able and willing to work after retirement, but the problem comes in finding jobs.

Finding substitute activities Many opportunities are available for older people who are willing to work on a volunteer basis in the church or community. The church leader can make these needs known and can encourage the retired peson to keep active.

While older people are still willing to serve, money is often a problem. For this reason, the church and other parts of society might consider ways in which people can receive at least a small honorarium for their volunteer work. This may be a wise expenditure of the Lord's money.

The married woman

In spite of the joys of being a homemaker, a woman's work is difficult and frequently unappreciated. For the housewife who has had a good education and has enjoyed a short career in nursing, teaching, office work or some other field, the role of changing diapers, mopping floors, and wiping noses is not very exciting work. Women who are homemakers need at times to be encouraged in their labors. They must realize that along with the joys and frustrations of being a housewife, they have the responsibility of molding young lives and maintaining a stable home. This is surely one of the most significant responsibilities that God gives.

The handicapped

A person's physical abilities and intelligence have an important influence on his vocational choice and adjustment. For the individual with a severe physical disability or for the person with below-average mental ability, there is a drastic limitation in the number of available jobs. Even when he finds a position, the handicapped person has adjustment problems that the rest of us do not face. The follower of Christ cannot ignore the lame, the blind or the otherwise disabled person.

THE CHURCH LEADER'S ROLE

Since most church leaders have no special expertise in this field, it is easy to conclude that the problems of vocational counseling should be left to someone better trained. Books on pastoral counseling often overlook this topic, failing to emphasize that the church leader can, in fact, make an important contribution to the vocational decisions of his congregation. Since he knows the family and since he – unlike most professionals – realizes the importance of God's will in vocational choice, the church leader is able to give special help.[7] In addition to more traditional vocational guidance, he can give spiritual counsel, provide information about church-related occupations, and write good letters of recommendation.

Spiritual guidance

When Jeremiah was called to be a prophet, he learned that there had been a divine plan for his life even before he was born (Jeremiah 1:5). The same was true for John the Baptist whose life work was described in detail prior to the time of his conception (Luke 1:13-17). Whether or not God has a similar plan for every life today is a debatable issue. All Christians agree, however, that God expects His followers to yield their whole lives to Him (Romans 12:1) and to serve Him faithfully (Psalm 2:11; Colossians 3:23-24; Hebrews 9:14). To do this we have been given different gifts, abilities and responsibilities (Romans 12:3-8; 1 Corinthians 12), and it is our duty to develop and use them in the best way possible.

In counseling on these issues, it is important to recognize that the first step in finding God's will for us is to *want* it. Too often we decide what we want – vocationally and otherwise – and then go to God in prayer, seeking a divine stamp of approval. "I'll go where you want me to go, dear Lord," we sing, "but with the following conditions . . ." Once we have completely committed ourselves and our careers to Christ, we must then *expect* that He will lead. The Scriptures assure us that God will guide in the decisions of life (Psalm 48:14; 73:24; Proverbs 3:5-6;

John 16:13a), but often we ignore these promises. We assume instead that God is playing some kind of a hide-and-seek game, telling us that He expects us to serve, but making it next to impossible for us to discover where and how.

Finally, it is necessary to *recognize that God guides in a variety of ways.* Rarely today, if ever, does He speak to people as He did to Saul on the road to Damascus. Instead, He apparently directs through Scripture, through our intellectual abilities, and through the circumstances of life. In making a career choice, for example, if we have completely yielded ourselves to God and are expecting Him to lead, we can then move ahead confidently, using every available resource, including the broad guidelines of Scripture, psychological test results, occupational information, the recommendations of counselors, the availability or non-availability of jobs and educational opportunities, and our own personal evaluation of the situation.

Sometimes a counselee must be reminded that, unlike us, God isn't always in a hurry. He does not always reveal His will when we want it, nor does He always show us the whole divine plan at once. Abraham packed his possessions and moved his whole family in response to the divine command to move, even though he "went out, not knowing where he was to go" (Hebrews 11:8, *RSV*). Many people today realize from personal experience that God still leads men in small steps.

Counseling concerning church vocations

Although all Christians are called to serve Christ, we are not all called to the same vocation. The body of Christ is composed of various occupational groups and nothing in Scripture suggests that professional missionaries, ordained ministers, seminary professors, or other "full-time Christian workers" are somehow more spiritual because of their church-related occupations. Surely God wants some people to be businessmen, secretaries, professional people, laborers, farmers, servicemen, or housewives. These people are also members of the body of Christ (1 Corinthians 12). They serve where they are and have a witness in areas which might be inaccessible to the professional churchman. In the New Testament, when a man became a Christian, he committed his life to Christ, but there was no expectation that he would automatically leave his occupation and become a pastor or traveling missionary.

Having acknowledged this, we must also recognize that God calls some men and women to church-related occupations. As they contemplate careers, these people will want to discuss their ideas with a person who is in the field being considered. The pastor, Christian education director, chaplain, minister of music, missionary, evangelist, seminary professor, or other church worker can provide firsthand information about his work. Unlike many other professionals, the church worker can more easily demonstrate by example what he does and he can invite the counselee to "get the feel" of the ministry by participating in a limited fashion.

In counseling concerning church vocations it is important to remember that we cannot always be certain of God's will for someone else's life. We can describe the various opportunities available and help the counselee in his deliberations, but he is the one who, under God, must make the final decisions. Of course, there is a real temptation to pressure someone to enter the ministry. The need is so immense, the shortage of good personnel is so acute, the satisfaction of guiding someone into the ministry is so great, that it is easy to push a person into a field to which he is neither called nor attracted.[8]

Writing letters of recommendation

The writing of good letters of recommendation is a laborious and time-consuming task, but it is a valuable way for the church leader to help others in their vocational planning. Many businesses and schools now send out forms in which the respondent can make his recommendation by checking from the several alternatives that are listed. This simplifies the task, but even the forms often leave a space for "further comments," and sometimes one might also want to include a letter with the form.

Instead of passing off these requests as a necessary nuisance, they should be taken seriously. In completing a form or writing a letter, remember that you have a responsibility to the applicant (it is best for him in the long run if we are honest - even if that prevents his application from being accepted), to the institution that seeks the information (as Christians we should not undermine their goal of getting capable people), to yourself and the name on the letterhead of your paper (it is of no credit to you if you "heartily recommend" someone who shouldn't be recommended), and to the Christ whom you follow.

Here is a real challenge for the church: to prepare people for a fluctuating world of work, to help them adjust to the changes, and to give them guidance as they seek to serve God in both their vocations and leisure-time activities.

5

Special Counseling Situations

No two counseling situations are ever exactly the same. However, there *are* similarities in counseling problems, and here we describe six special situations.

COUNSELING THE MENTALLY ILL

Very often people who are mentally ill differ little from the rest of us except for the fact that the problems of life have become so overwhelming that it is difficult for them to behave or think efficiently. Frequently there are discouragements, anxiety, confusion, a sense of failure, a loss of self-esteem, and feelings of frustration because one has succumbed to the pressure of life.

Counseling with the disturbed individual

The church leader faces four important challenges as he works with emotionally disturbed people and their families. *First,* he can recognize the signs of emotional turmoil. Even when the symptoms are obvious, family members are sometimes reluctant to face the reality of the situation and to encourage their relative to seek professional help. This is especially true if the family harbors the view that mental illness is a disgrace. Then the symptoms are explained away as a "temporary upset" or the result of "working too hard." The family clings to the hope that, given time, the unusual behavior will disappear. In many cases this does happen, but more often the problems get worse and treatment is simply delayed. While encouraging the church leader to be alert in looking for symptoms, we would also caution against being too quick to see problems where none exist. The pastor who sees a psychotic in every pew will soon lose his effectiveness as a counselor.

Second, the counselor can help the disturbed person get competent treatment. Sometimes the church leader himself can do an effective job of counseling, but at other times he will want to encourage referral to a mental health professional or treatment center.

In considering referral, try to determine where the counselee can get the best possible help. Sometimes a private psychiatrist or psychologist will give the most effective treatment, but at other times it may be better to consider the psychiatric ward in a general hospital, a local mental health center, a private psychiatric hospital, or a nearby state or provincial hospital. In making this decision, the financial means of the family, the seriousness of the problem, and the known effectiveness of the various referral sources should all be considered, along with the general *welfare* of the patient and his family.

If commitment to a psychiatric hospital seems advisable, it is best if the patient agrees to this voluntarily, supported by the encouragement of the family and pastor. But if the patient is severely disturbed and unwilling to get help, legal commitment may be necessary. Admission to a mental hospital is often accompanied by considerable anxiety, loneliness and fear. The counselor must help all involved to accept the reality of the situation, encouraging everyone to work together so the treatment will be successful.[1]

The *third role* of the church leader in working with the severely disturbed is to the hospitalized. The patient who is confused, lonely or hurt can be helped immeasurably by visits from concerned friends, but often church leaders are reluctant to visit. Perhaps they don't know what to expect when they call on a mental patient, or they are afraid of being unwelcome or are unsure of what to say. A good ground rule is to call on the mental patient as you would call on anybody else. Keep the visit brief; be cheerful and understanding; use prayer and the Scriptures (but keep this short and avoid scriptural passages which are likely to be misinterpreted by a patient whose thinking may be distorted); be encouraging, but avoid making promises that you cannot keep or taking sides if the patient is complaining or critical. According to one hospital chaplain, the mere fact that you stay for a while and return for subsequent visits, "can be one of the most constructive contributions to the patient's recovery."[2]

Following hospitalization, the church leader has his *fourth* opportunity: helping the patient during the time of rehabilitation. Many pressures of family and community living which may have contributed to the "breakdown" in the first place are still around when the patient leaves the hospital. In addition there is, for some, embarrassment over being an "ex-mental patient." Church leaders, as well as members of the congregation, must learn to accept the former patient and welcome him back into the church. He should be welcomed back, encouraged, and treated as any other person who has been hospitalized.[3]

Counseling with the family

When a relative develops mental illness, many families feel this is a major crisis. The patient's unusual behavior, the social stigma which still surrounds "mental illness," and the necessary readjustments when a relative is hospitalized, all put pressure on the family unit. Often there are confusion, anxiety and misunderstanding. For some families the crisis pulls everyone together, but for others the situation causes disintegration.

The church leader can help the disturbed patient's family in several ways, according to Clinebell.[4]

1 He can help them to recognize and accept the fact that the person is, indeed, emotionally disturbed.

2 He can help the family and the patient in finding competent treatment.

3 He can give encouragement and help the family towards increased dependence on God. He should maintain a counseling relationship which informs, permits expression of feelings, and encourages discussion of "why God would permit something like this."

4 Relatives can be helped to discuss and accept their feelings about mental illness in the family. They could be encouraged to make hospital visits – and guided as they prepare to receive the patient on his return from hospital.

COUNSELING THE PHYSICALLY ILL

When a person becomes physically ill much more is involved than the malfunctioning of his body and the development of physical symptoms. Sickness brings, in addition, a number of psychological reactions such as anxiety, frustration and uncertainty both in the patient and his family, and may also lead to financial strain. The *transition period* from health to sickness may be sudden (as with a heart attack) or very gradual (as with cancer). Sometimes the person does not want to face his symptoms and avoids seeing a doctor in the hope that the physical problems will clear up spontaneously or in response to home remedies. Persisting symptoms, or the sudden onset of serious illness eventually make denial impossible, but it still takes time to adjust to the realization that one is sick, and may remain so for a long time.

In the *treatment period,* the person faces his symptoms and gives himself over to medical treatment, but this can also be a time of difficulty. In addition to the physical discomfort there is often fear of the unknown. "What is really wrong with me?" the patient wonders. "Will the doctors make an accurate diagnosis?" "Will we be able to pay for all of this?" "How will the family get along while I'm sick?" Further conflicts may arise as the patient is faced with hospitalization and dependence upon others after his accustomed independence.

In the *convalescence period* the person and his family slowly make the transition from sickness back to health. This can be a smooth process but it may also be fraught with difficulties.

Counseling the patient and the family

When He was on earth, Jesus spent a great deal of time ministering to the sick and, as His followers, we should be grateful for the privilege of doing likewise. The church leader can be an encouragement to both the patient and his family during their time of crisis, and a reminder that the Great Physician is aware and concerned about the physical problems of His children. We can pray for and with the people involved, encourage the ventilation of fears and frustrations, guide in their thinking about why God permitted this situation to arise, and point to relevant passages of Scripture.

Counseling when a child is sick

When a child becomes sick, the church leader is presented with a unique counseling situation. Like adults, children feel pain, fear the unknown, dislike the strangeness of the hospital, and do not want to be separated from loved ones. They do not understand what is happening, why they are suffering, or why people in white clothes stick them with needles or give bad-tasting medicines. For many children, hospitalization is interpreted as parental rejection or even punishment for past behavior. The church leader has a ministry both to the child and to the family – especially the parents. How one counsels with a child will depend largely on the age and level of understanding, but children should always be reassured and not deceived. By supportive counseling with the parents we can help the child indirectly, because when he senses that his parents are calm he feels greater assurance. However, often it is difficult for parents to feel this calmness; as every parent knows, there is nothing more heart-rending than to look into the face of a little sick child who doesn't understand. Parents often appreciate support from a Christian friend who is willing to listen, encourage, and simply "be present."[5] In addition, the comfort of prayer and the Scriptures should be an important part of a ministry of counseling with parents, and grandparents as well.

COUNSELING THE DYING

Death has always been surrounded by fear, anxiety and unhappiness. Even Christians who believe that to be absent from the body is to be present with the Lord (2 Corinthians 5:8), shrink from thoughts of death and are uncomfortable in its presence.[6]

In an attempt to study how people react when faced with their own death, four theological students approach a psychiatrist several years ago at the University of Chicago Hospital. After first meeting considerable resistance from hospital personnel who wanted the patients to be "left alone," the psychiatrist and her seminary students began interviewing terminally ill patients. Their findings have been published in a very interesting book and shed considerable light on the attitudes of the dying and how these people can be counseled.[7]

Understanding the dying

On the basis of carefully conducted psychiatric interviews with over one hundred terminally ill patients, Dr. Kubler-

Ross has defined five stages that people go through as they approach death:

First stage: denial and isolation "No, it can't happen to me" is the initial reaction of the patient when he learns or suspects that his sickness is terminal. This denial is a defense used by all patients, especially at the beginning of their illness. None of us wants to believe that our death is imminent, and it helps people to handle the shock if they can periodically deny the truth of the diagnosis.

Second stage: anger Patients can't keep denying the truth forever, and slowly they come to acknowledge the fact that they are dying. Such a realization is accompanied by anger and resentment. "Why me?" they wonder. "Why couldn't it have been somebody who is old or alone or of no use to society?" Often this frustration and anger lead the patient to be highly demanding and highly critical of hospital personnel. Sometimes this even results in turning against loved ones, criticism of the pastor who visits, and anger against God. When this happens, the family members are often surprised and bewildered. They take the verbal attack personally, failing to realize that the patient's anger is really irrational - but normal - lashing out in response to a frustrating situation. At this time the patient needs understanding from loved ones rather than hurt or indignant argument in response to his outburst.

Third stage: bargaining Little children who don't get their way by throwing a tantrum often resort next to a charming manner in which they try to persuade others to give them favors. The terminally ill person tends to act in a similar manner. Following the period of anger there is a time of bargaining for longer life or freedom from pain. "God, give me a little longer," they may ask, "and I'll serve You faithfully for the rest of my life."

Fourth stage: depression As the illness lingers on, discouragement sets in. This is commonly of two types: As its name implies, reactive depression comes as a reaction against the illness and its effects. The second type, preparatory depression, is really a form of grief as the patient anticipates the future. He may be a believer who looks forward to the "far better" time after death, but he is concerned about the loved ones who will remain and perhaps experience great difficulties when he is gone.

Fifth stage: acceptance Few patients keep resisting to the end; if the illness has been long, most eventually reach a stage of acceptance. This should not be mistaken for a happy stage. It is almost void of feelings. . . . This is also the time during which the *family* needs usually more help, understanding, and support than the patient himself.[8]

The patient may not want to talk, but he is comforted in knowing that he is not forgotten, even when the end is near.

Hope There are broad individual differences in the way people approach death. The five stages may not be seen in everyone, especially if the length of illness is short. The approach to death may differ if one has a strong assurance that he will soon be with Christ. Regardless of the religious convictions, however, almost all terminally ill patients show at least some hope: "I might still get better." Dr. Kubler-Ross concluded, "if a patient stops expressing hope, it is usually a sign of imminent death."[9]

Counseling the dying

The place to begin in any ministry to the dying is with our own attitudes. Most of us – including Christians – do not like to think about death. Perhaps many believers unconsciously expect that they will be among those who will avoid death and go directly to be with Christ (1 Thessalonians 4:16-17). Whatever the reason, we frequently avoid discussing our own death and, in so doing, we leave a number of important decisions for the surviving spouse to make during the first hours of grief. Medical personnel, family members, and even pastors or other church leaders tend to avoid the dying patient, perhaps because we feel uncomfortable in his presence. Even when a chaplain or pastor calls, there is frequently a tendency to read a passage of Scripture and lead in prayer, but to avoid all reference to death or to the needs and concerns of the dying.[10] A careful consideration of the biblical statements about death, thinking about one's own death, and a discussion of funeral arrangements with one's family need not be an unhealthful dwelling on morbid events. Instead, it is an exercise which will make death easier when it comes and will enable us to more openly and comfortably discuss the subject when we counsel with the dying and their families. Such counseling must be characterized by the counselor's/pastor's availability and genuine concern. Sometimes the counselor can help in the discussion of practical plans for the future, and he should encourage those involved to recognize and talk about the guilt that is so often present at the time of death.

Kubler-Ross suggests that most people know intuitively when they are dying, and for this reason it is usually best to face the reality of the situation openly. This frees both patient and family to discuss the future and to better communicate with each other.

COUNSELING THE GRIEVING

Even when death comes at the end of a long terminal illness, grief is hard burden to bear. It involves a number of emotions, including sorrow, despair, anxiety, guilt, loneliness, anger, confusion, futility, and an over-bearing sense of loss as someone who has long been part of us is now taken away for the rest of our lives.

Usually grief begins with a *period of shock*. When we learn that a loved one has died, there is often dazed disbelief, sometimes accompanied by physical symptoms such as nausea, faintness, stomach pains or throbbing headaches. Before the time of the funeral, the mourner has usually entered a *period of intense grief*. Copious weeping, intense yearning for the lost person, self-condemnation because of past times when we were inconsiderate, and preoccupation with memories of the deceased are all common in the weeks following death. Christians may frequently pray and search the Scriptures - asking the question, "Why?" Later, perhaps after a month or two, the mourner slowly moves into a long *period of readjustment*. Life with its challenges must be picked up again but without the departed loved one being present. This includes a return to work, a resumption of normal activities, and some involvement in social affairs.

Needs of the grieving

The need for support from others At a time of grief it is important to have others, includ-ing people from the church, who can be present or available to listen, share and help.

The need to accept the reality of the loss The intellectual knowledge that someone has died as well as the emotional acceptance of this fact are often two different issues. The mourner must go through the painful process of accepting the reality of the loss – a process which usually takes several months. To do this there is often a need to talk about the departed one, to relive past memories, and to remind oneself that the loss has actually occurred.

The need to express sorrow When He arrived at the home of Mary and Martha following the death of their brother, Jesus openly wept (John 11:35). This may seem strange when we consider that Jesus knew in advance that Lazarus would be restored to life (John 11:11-15), but by His example the Lord showed that the expression of sorrow is quite appropriate even among those who knew that the departed one is "with Christ; which is far better" (Philippians 1:23). Therefore, the church leader must permit and encourage the outpouring of feelings, for this is a necessary part of grieving - for believers and nonbelievers alike.

The need to verbalize hostility and guilt Books and articles on grief make frequent reference to the anger and hostility that are often experienced by grief-stricken persons.[11]

Sometimes the anger is directed toward other people or toward God. Such anger may seem irrational, but it is a commonly observed reaction to frustration. Anger directed inward toward oneself is also common. This is really self-condemnation for what was said or not said, done or not done, while the dead person was alive.

The need to establish relationships The grieving person must find others who can provide the security and satisfaction that the former relationship provided. This is a difficult and time-consuming process which can be accompanied by guilt if the mourner feels that in building new friendship he is also being unfaithful to the deceased.

Counseling the grieving

The pastor and members of the congregation play at least three major roles in counseling with the sorrowing. First, they *bring the comfort of the Scriptures*. The Bible pictures death as a great gain for the believer and something to be welcomed (Philippians 1:21). By His own death and resurrection Christ overpowered death so that the believer is assured of everlasting life in the presence of the risen Lord (John 3:16; 14:1-3; 1 Corinthians 15:54-57; 1 Thessalonians 4:13-18). For those who mourn, Jesus promised comfort (Matthew 5:4), and He described the Holy Spirit as "the Comforter" (John 14:26), who would be present in times of grief. Over the centuries great numbers of believers have felt this "peace of God, which passeth all understanding" (Philippians 4:7). Such a divine comfort is supplemented by the comfort that believers show for one another in times of sorrow. Only Christ gives real peace, and we should remind one another of this in times of sorrow (1 Thessalonians 4:18).

The funeral is a ceremony for the living – not for the dead. In the first place, it forces people to face the painful truth that death has, in fact, occurred. A memorial service without the body being present may be much easier to bear, but it does little to bring home the harsh reality that must be faced eventually. In addition, the funeral is an opportunity for friends to express their concern and support for the bereaved. For Christians, the funeral is also an opportunity to worship and give witness of the hope that is within.

In ministering to the grieving, the church leader can *help in the planning for a funeral.* (Ideally, of course, Christians should think about this before they die.) He can help the family to make decisions about the type and cost of the coffin, the place of the funeral (church or funeral home), and the details of the service. He can lead in a worship experience which "strengthens and undergirds," which expresses the comfort of Christ and the concern of friends, but which also helps the mourner to accept the reality of death.

The third role of the church leader is to *guide during the period of readjustment.* When the funeral is over, the flowers have wilted, and the relatives have gone home, the months which follow are often very lonely and painful. It is here that the concerned Christian tries to be available to bring the comfort of friends and the Scriptures, and to guide as the mourner works to satisfy the needs outlined in the preceding pages.

Death and the young child

After completing a study of almost 1,000 bereaved people, Gorer, an English writer, concluded that the death of a child is "the most distressing and long-lasting of all griefs. . . . In such a case it seems to be literally true, and not a figure of speech, that the parents never get over it."[12] That life should end for a little child with so much potential is a painful realization, even if we expect to see him again in eternity (2 Samuel 12:23).

It can also be difficult to explain to a child that someone whom he loves has died. The way in which this is presented and the words that are used depend largely on the child's age and level of understanding. For children of all ages it is important to openly discuss the death and to give reassurance that the surviving child is loved and will be cared for, no matter what are the circumstances.[13]

COUNSELING THE PHYSICALLY DISABLED

During His earthly ministry, Jesus showed a deep concern for the physically disabled. He ministered to the blind, the deaf, the lame, and others who were physically infirm, and many of His followers did likewise.

A physically disabled person is one whose body has a defect or impairment which partially hinders or interferes with the person's ability to function normally in the society. The person with paralyzed legs, for example, has a part of his body that is not functioning. Because of this, he cannot walk normally and must remain confined to a wheelchair. Notice, however, that he is only partially handicapped. He can still think, use his arms, see, hear and talk. This illustrates an important truth about the disabled person. While there are things which he *cannot* do, there are also things which he *can do*.[14] This is important to remember in counseling.

Understanding the disabled

People who are disabled from birth apparently adjust smoothly to their condition. It is always frustrating to overcome a physical disability, but those who are born with a defect cope with it from birth. They do not know what it feels like to have the body functioning normally, and thus don't miss what they have never known.[15]

Undoubtedly the situation is more difficult when a person is disabled later in life. Fink has identified four stages that such people go through: *shock* when the disability first occurs; *retreat* behind a number of psychological defenses which enable one to temporarily avoid facing the full impact of the situation; *acknowledgment* in which the person slowly faces the almost overwhelming implications of the disability; and *adaptation* in which the person adjusts to his disabled condition.[16]

The physically disabled person must make a number of psychological adjustments that those with a more "normal" physique can avoid. For example, he must adjust to being different. Little children look at him with open curiosity while adults glance at him in a more subtle way, avoid him, or sometimes treat him with scorn. Like everyone else, the disabled person wants to be treated with respect and to feel that he is a worthy individual, but this is a difficult goal to reach. The author remembers vividly a mildly disabled young lady of thirty-one who approached him after a church service one night. "You're a psychologist," she said with tears in her eyes. "Tell me why I've never had a date. I want to get married like anyone else."

Counseling the disabled

The first task in counseling the physically disabled is to convey acceptance. We must treat the counselee as a person of worth who has characteristics that are desirable, feelings that need to be expressed, needs that must be met, frustrations that must be overcome. If he wants to *appear* accepting, the counselor must really *be* accepting. If he cannot be accepting, he needs to take an honest look at his own attitudes and perhaps discuss them with some confidant.

As we accept the handicapped person, we must seek to help him accept himself, to realistically evaluate his limitations, to overcome obstacles when he can, and to function as efficiently as possible with his limitations. He must come to recognize that, regardless of his handicap, he is an individual whom God loves and whom Christ came to redeem. We must guide him in his spiritual growth, helping him to find and follow God's will for his life. Also, we must be willing to discuss questions of "Why?" and help him accept the difficulties in his life.

The church leader is not the only person involved in working with the handicapped. Parents (who often need understanding and encouragement themselves as they cope with their feelings and the special demands of their handicapped children) physicians, teachers, vocational counselors and others must work together to help the disabled. Members of the congregation must be encouraged to take an interest in the handicapped, to accept them as people, to help them get to the church, and to guide in their spiritual, emotional, social and vocational development.

COUNSELING THE DISADVANTAGED OR THOSE FROM MINORITY GROUPS

Regardless of whom we classify as disadvantaged, it should be recognized from the start that counseling with and ministering to people of other ethnic and socio-economic groups is very difficult. To counsel with any disadvantaged group we must expect to be rejected at first and treated as a potential enemy. We must have patience, Christian love, understanding, acceptance, and complete freedom from any holier-than-thou attitudes. In spite of the difficulties, however, we cannot fulfill the Great Commission while ignoring the disadvantaged nearby. Every church leader should consider how his congregation, if not he himself, can have some impact on this difficult mission field which may be literally around the corner.

THE QUESTION OF "WHY?"

Throughout this chapter and earlier in this book we have mentioned that people whom a church leader counsels frequently ask "Why?" Why do I have this problem? Why did God let this happen? Why didn't it happen to someone else? Why do ministers say that God is loving and good when He permits such sadness and misery? These are difficult questions which should be pondered before they have to be answered in a counseling session. They are also theological questions which are out of the domain of psychology.

In the Bible the answers to "why" questions are not always clear. We *do* know that when God permits or brings about some stressful situation, He does so for a good purpose (Romans 8:28). It may be to produce patience (James 1:3), humility (2 Corinthians 12:7-10), or a deeper dependence on God (2 Corinthians 1:8-9). Sometimes it is an expression of divine love for us and, even though we may feel miserable at the time, the Scriptures describe those whom the Lord chastens as "blessed" (Psalm 94:12; Proverbs 3:11-12; Revelation 3:19).

In counseling, the Christian leader can point the *counselee* to those passages of Scripture which deal with suffering (see especially 1 Peter and Job). He can guide as the counselee ventilates his feelings and seeks to find answers in the Scriptures. But he can also point to the example of Job. Though he suffered through a series of setbacks that would have overwhelmed most of us, and though his counselors only added to the problems, Job was never told why it all happened. God has a purpose (Job 1-2), but Job never knew what this was.* In many cases the same is true today. So long as we live on earth, the ways of God are often beyond our comprehension (Romans 11:33). Even Christ simply "placed His hopes in God, the righteous Judge" (1 Peter 2:23).

* See suggestions for further readings on page 182.

III

Problems in Counseling

6

Guilt

As part of my training to become a psychologist I spent several months working in a clinic for physically handicapped children. Each morning a number of parents would come to this clinic with their disabled children and the family would participate in two days of intensive diagnostic examinations. A pediatrician, orthopedic surgeon, child psychiatrist, physical therapist, social worker, and clinical psychologist would, at different times, meet with the parents and the child and then meet together as a professional team to pool their knowledge and discuss how the young patient could be helped.

One morning a mother came into my office and gave her appraisal of why she had a mentally and physically handicapped daughter.

"It is punishment from God," the lady stated.

"I was a missionary in Africa but when I came home on my first furlough, I met a man, fell in love, and got married. My husband is a fine Christian and he is good to me as well, but he never felt called to the mission field. Because I never went back God has punished me with this sick child."

The woman who sat across the desk was obviously plagued with guilt. Her whole life was characterized by feelings of remorse because she had not remained a missionary.

Guilt has been described as the place where psychology and religion meet. Probably there is no other topic which is of equal interest to both theologians and psychologists. Dr. Ernest Jones, a psychoanalyst who wrote a three-volume biography of Freud, once described guilt as the most difficult and the most important problem in the whole realm of psychology. Almost all of man's troubles, Jones believed, can be traced to our inner feeling of guilt.

The meaning and prevalence of guilt

Guilt arises when we have consciously done something wrong: when we have violated ethical, legal, moral, or religious standards. Often, but not always, guilt is accompanied by feelings of regret and self-condemnation. Sometimes guilt arises because we have done something wrong and wish we hadn't, while at other times we feel guilt because we failed to do something we knew to be right. The Episcopal prayer book states it concisely in the prayer of confession: "We have done those things which we ought not to have done and we have left undone those things which we ought to have done and there is no health in us." Most of us fail in the way of that prayer every day. We say an unkind word, we procrastinate, we get too busy to spend time with our families, we fail to meet an obligation, we have some immoral thought, or we ignore our conscience and deliberately sin. All of this brings guilt, often accompanied by feelings of remorse and self-criticism.

But even if we have no reason to feel guilty in ourselves, other people have a way of stirring it up within us. It is a very useful way to manipulate other people, to get our children (or our parents) to do what we want. The teenager who complains, "Everyone else is doing it . . ." often wishes his parents to feel guilty because of their stubborn resistance. Pressured parents sometimes yield in order to relieve their "guilt." The husband who yells to his wife, "I drink because you nag all the time," pushes the blame on her and tries to make her feel guilty, thus relieving himself of responsibility for his own actions. The pastor who threatens to resign because people don't go along with his programmes or come to his services may be manipulating them to feel sorry for him, to feel guilty, and, therefore, inclined to change their behavior. Children attempt this too. Recently our four-year old wanted some candy and was distressed when her mother said no. "If you don't give it to me," my daughter pouted, "I'll be very unhappy and I'll cry." This attempt to make her mother feel guilty and give in was unsuccessful, but I wondered where she had learned that making others feel guilty is a good way to manipulate them into doing what you want. (I would like to think she learned the tactic from neighborhood children, but I have a suspicion she may have learned it from me!)

Types of guilt

Guilt is so widespread in our society, so common an experience, and so often mentioned in theological and psychological literature, that several types have been identified. These can be divided into two categories: **objective guilt** and **subjective guilt**. Objective guilt exists apart from our feelings. Here the person has broken some legal standard and he is guilty whether he feels it or not. Subjective guilt is a feeling or inner experience of remorse because of one's actions.

Objective guilt is further divided into three types.

First, *social guilt.* Here the individual is guilty because he has broken a law or accepted a rule that most people around him obey. When I drive at 80 kph in a 40 kph zone I break the law. I may or may not feel guilty, but if I happen to pass a policeman I will probably be stopped and given a fine or court summons. Sometimes social guilt comes because we have broken an unwritten law. If I engage in an act that, according to those around me, wrongs another person or group of people, I am guilty of harming a relationship with others. I may criticize someone unkindly, ignore my children, pass by a person in need, or gossip maliciously. In doing these things I may have broken no legal written laws, and I may not even feel bad, but I have violated the social expectations of my society. Thus, I am guilty, after engaging in an act that puts a barrier between other people and myself.

The second type of objective guilt might be called *psychological guilt.* This arises because I have done something which goes against my own personal standards. The Apostle Paul discussed this in Romans 14 and 1 Corinthians 10. There was nothing legally wrong with eating meat that had been offered to idols and for most people there was nothing morally wrong with it. For some, however, this was a sinful act; to consume that meat would have produced guilt in the eater because he had ignored his inner standards and conscience. In a more modern setting, the student who decides that he should read four books every month may experience guilt if he does not meet this goal. Psychological guilt in this student comes only because he has not reached his own very personal and private goal.

A third type of objective guilt arises from our relationship with God. Sometimes called *ontological* or *theological guilt*, it refers to our standing before God. According to the Bible, all men have sinned and have come short of the glory of God (Romans 3:23). We have all disobeyed God, ignored His voice at times, and selfishly refused to trust Him. We are all guilty of breaking our relationship with God, even though we might not feel such guilt.

Most of us would feel uncomfortable if we had broken social law (social guilt), violated our conscience (psychological guilt), or deliberately ignored God (ontological guilt). However it is possible to do all of these things and not feel even a twinge of guilt. The hardened criminal may murder and not feel anything. Millions of people, including Christians, forget God everyday and sin against Him. While these people are guilty before God they feel no sense of guilt because of their actions.

The matter of feelings brings us to the second broad category of guilt, **subjective guilt.**

When we talk about guilt, most of us refer to the subjective feeling that people so often experience when they do wrong or have unacceptable (to them) thoughts and wishes. The person who cheats on his income tax, the Christian who misses church service, or the wife who thinks unkind thoughts about her in-laws, all may feel a great sense of self-blame and humiliation.

These subjective feelings of guilt may be appropriate or inappropriate. Appropriate guilt feelings arise when we have broken a law and feel remorse in proportion to the seriousness of our action. Inappropriate guilt feelings are those which appear to be out of proportion to the seriousness of our action. Some people, for example, feel nothing even when they act in a way which seriously violates the law, goes against their own moral standards, and is a sin against God. This lack of guilt feeling is inappropriate, highly unusual and might even be classified as neurotic. At the opposite extreme are those people who are overwhelmed by feelings of guilt. They feel guilt very strongly even when they have done something which others consider to be minor.

I once counseled a lady who for many years had taken care of an elderly and demanding father-in-law. One day, in the midst of anger, the lady told her father-in-law, "Shut up!" For days afterward this woman worried, chided herself and felt condemned because she had spoken so harshly to an old man. Also at times those who express constant guilt feelings are playing a game with themselves, saying they feel guilty about one thing when really it is something else that is bothering them. They may, for example, feel great remorse about missing a church service but whether they recognize it or not, they really are guilty of something else - ignoring God in their lives.

Causes of guilt

How does guilt arise? In the first place guilt comes about because our conscience bothers us. Most psychologists think of the conscience as an inner experience of right and wrong that develops as we grow up. By listening to the teachings of our parents or teachers and by watching others, we learn what they say is right or wrong, good or bad, moral or immoral. Soon the standards of others become our standards. They become part of us and thus when our actions are at odds with these standards we feel uncomfortable and guilty.

Although psychologists all agree that the conscience

is acquired, scriptural evidence suggests that standards of right and wrong may also be inborn (Romans 2:14, 15), God apparently has written some standards within the hearts of men: when we violate these standards we are guilty.

This brings us to a second reason for feeling guilt: supernatural influences. We know that the Holy Spirit convicts men of their sin, speaks to us about what is true and right, and reminds us of the teachings of Jesus (John 16:8, 13). Unlike other religions, Christianity gives us a perfect person, Jesus Christ, who is a standard by which we mold our lives. When we ignore or fall short of this standard the Holy Spirit reminds us of it.

But the Holy Spirit is not the only supernatural influence that may bring about feelings of guilt. Satan also accuses us (Job 1:9-11; Revelation 12:10). He also arouses guilt feelings and makes us feel uncomfortable, especially if we are obedient to God. Therefore, while guilt feelings are sometimes healthy and beneficial (when they are aroused by the Holy Spirit), at other times they are unhealthy and harmful (when they are aroused by satanic forces). How do we tell the difference? God's standard of right and wrong is clearly outlined in the Bible and we can be sure that the Holy Spirit never directs us to do something contrary to the written Word of God (1 John 4).

The consequences of guilt

When we think of guilt most of us probably think of something undesirable. While this is often true, we should realize that guilt and guilt feelings can also be desirable. If we never became aware of ontological guilt, for example, we might never see the need for a Savior. If we never had any guilt feelings we might be more inclined to act in ways which would harm other people and harm ourselves. Guilt and guilt feelings, therefore, are not always bad. Sometimes they are constructive and helpful.

Still, guilt feelings often influence us adversely - especially when we rationalize guilt and pretend it does not exist. We do this when we make up excuses to explain our guilt away: "Of course I cheated on my income tax!" We say to ourselves, "but everybody does it." Or, "certainly I went over the speed limit but there weren't any other cars around and they probably expect most people to do a little over the posted speed anyhow." Equally common is the tendency to pass the buck by blaming someone else for our guilt-producing behavior. Adam blamed Eve who in turn blamed the serpent. Hitler blamed the Jews for his difficulties and at the end of his life wrote, "It is true that neither I nor anybody else in Germany wanted war in 1939. It was wanted and provoked exclusively by those international politicians who either came of Jewish stock or worked for Jewish interests. After all my efforts toward disarmament, posterity cannot place the responsibility for this war on me."[1] This also happens when we blame our friends for their bad influence on us or we deny we are responsible for our actions since so much behavior is determined by our past experiences, or the influence of our parents. (More and more people, it seems, are claiming they cannot be held responsible for their actions since they are the helpless victims of unhealthy childhood experiences.)

When we push guilt from our conscious awareness, we can be sure it will come back to haunt us in other ways. *Denied guilt*, for example, *often causes physical illness*. The mere effort of keeping the guilt out of one's mind can put a strain on the body and cause it to break down. It is also quite possible that guilty people punish themselves unconsciously by getting sick. This may sound ridiculous until you recognize that according to several estimates, between 50 and 75 percent of all patients who go to a medical doctor are suffering from physical ill- nesses that are emotionally caused. If we are physically sick we get a lot of sympathy and almost nobody holds us responsible for our actions - including the actions that are causing the guilt.

Denied guilt can also cause depression. Here the person has done something for which he feels guilty but instead of facing his guilt he develops feelings of hopelessness, worthlessness, despair, and discouragement.

A third way denied guilt influences us is by causing self-destructive behavior. I once counseled with a very bright young man who had never succeeded in anything. As we talked it became apparent to me that he really didn't want to succeed. He was unconsciously sabotaging his own success in order to pay for some guilt he was trying to keep hidden. Perhaps you have heard of the flagellants in the Philippines. On Good Friday each year these men walk through the streets beating themselves with whips, literally tearing their backs to shreds. It would seem the individuals feel guilty and think they should punish themselves. Some writers have even suggested that accident proneness may characterize people who are unconsciously angry with themselves for past deeds.

Fourthly, denied guilt can cause neuroses. Often the guilty person develops what psychologists call an obsessive-compulsive neurosis in which the individual feels a compulsion to do something over and over again since such repetitious acts seem to help one to fight off guilt. Lady MacBeth's repetitious handwashing is a good example from Shakespeare. This neurosis also characterizes the behavior of many religious people. When a person feels he must rigidly attend every church service, serve on every committee and engage in every ritual, these may be unconscious attempts to ward off guilt feelings. For these people life becomes a great burden. Their religion becomes a list of dos and don'ts they never know the real joy that comes from a guilt-free Christ- centered life.

Dealing with guilt

For many years psychiatrists and psychologists have struggled with the problem of how people can be freed from guilt. One of the most common solutions has been to change our views of what is right or wrong. "Lower your standards," some psychologists say, "and learn to do as you please without feeling guilty." Such a solution has been widely accepted in our culture but since it only deals with guilt *feelings* (not objective guilt), it rarely works. Men today feel increasingly confused, discouraged, anxious, and guilty in spite of the lowering of moral standards. Guilt has to be handled in some other way.

Our whole legal system in this world is built on the assumption that the one who breaks the law must pay; all of the burdensome symptoms we have listed on guilt reflect attempts by men to pay for their guilty behavior. The Bible, however, tells us that Christ has already paid (1 Peter 3:18). It is because of Jesus Christ's death for our wrong-doing that we are able to deal with guilt permanently and effectively. To do so there are five basic and necessary steps.

1 **The first of these is repentance.** In the preceding pages we have avoided using the word "sin." The Bible is clear, however, in stating that men are sinners and that it is sin

which causes guilt and guilt feelings. To be free of guilt, we must recognize, as did the Psalmist King David, that whenever we do wrong we are really sinning against God who alone is sinless (Psalm 51:4). To overcome our guilt we must recognize that apart from God, no man can really do good and that our so-called righteous acts are really as acceptable to God as a pile of filthy rags (Isaiah 64:6). In short, we must be sincerely ashamed and sorry that we have sinned against a holy God.

2 **But there is more to removing guilt than feeling sorry for what we are and have done.** Some people spend their lives in self-debasement and still feel guilty. The second step in dealing with our guilt, therefore is *confession.* The Scriptures show us two kinds. First, there is confession of our sins to God. This step is necessary if we ever hope to experience forgiveness (1 John 1:9). This confession of specific sins should be a daily occurrence if we expect to be free from guilt and guilt feelings. In addition, the Scriptures also teach the importance of confession to other men. The writer of the book of James encourages this and so did Jesus when He instructed men to be reconciled to each other (James 5:16).

3 **This brings us to the third step in dealing with guilt, forgiveness.** When we confess, God forgives. This is a simple truth with profound implications for guilty man. But notice that we are not only to receive forgiveness, but we are to forgive others when they confess to us. The Lord's Prayer mentions this and in Matthew 18:21-23 we read of an occasion where Jesus discussed the issue at length. Some of us confess sin to God (and are forgiven by God) but don't feel forgiven. Might it be that our refusal to forgive others stands in the way of experiencing the relief

that otherwise would come?

It is also important that we forgive ourselves. Many of us are forgiven by God but go on feeling guilty because we have not forgiven ourselves. Perhaps these people don't really believe that God has forgiven or that He is able to forgive. Like the father who once brought his ailing son to Jesus, these people must honestly cry, "Lord, I believe; help thou mine unbelief" (Mark 9:23-25).

4 **The fourth step in dealing with guilt is summarized in the word restitution.** In the Bible we read about a man named Zacchaeus who, besides being a tax collector, was also a crook. One day Jesus met him and forgave him for his dishonesty. After Zacchaeus accepted the gift of forgiveness, he decided to pay back everything that he had stolen with interest. This paying back was not necessary in order for Zacchaeus to be forgiven but it grew out of his changed life (Luke 19:1-10).

According to the Bible, there is no need for men to pay or make restitution for their sins. In fact, we are not able to do this, which is why Christ paid instead. But when we realize that our sins are paid for and forgiven, it is natural that we should respond by giving to others and by making restitution as an act of worship and thanksgiving.

5 **The final step in dealing with guilt is changed behavior.** Like the woman taken in adultery we must go and sin no more (John 8:11). We must yield ourselves to the living Christ and commit ourselves to His service. We must count on Him for courage and strength to overcome guilt and to resist the temptations of the Devil. We must realize that even if we sin again, God has made provision to remove the guilt (1 John 2:1, 2).

To accept all of this is difficult. We have bodies that are subject to temptation and we know that too often we yield.

When we sin, there is little value in engaging in morbid introspection, in making excuses for our sins, or in hiding our guilt. Instead, we can confess our sin knowing that it will be forgiven and that the guilt will be removed because Christ died not for our sins only, "but for the sins of the whole world" (1 John 2:1, 2).

Sometimes we find that we are worrying and berating ourselves about minor sins while we ignore something major. Sometimes we sincerely want to rid ourselves of guilt but find that we have difficulty following the five steps that are outlined above. At such times we can often find help if we share our concerns and evaluate our guilt by talking with another person.

7

A Look at Inferiority

Shortly after the turn of the century a famous psychiatrist in Austria named Alfred Adler attempted to analyze the thinking of very young children.[1] He recognized that babies and toddlers are really very helpless creatures: they are smaller, less capable, less skilled, less successful, and less powerful than almost anyone else around. As a result, all children develop what Adler called feelings of inferiority. These feelings are not *all* bad since they motivate the child to overcome his deficiencies or inadequacies.

Adler reached a further conclusion. Little children, he decided, are not the only people who feel inferior; all of us feel inferior to some extent. To "be a human being," he once wrote, "means the possession of inferiority that is constantly spurring us on to greater achievements."[2] Feelings of inferiority and incompleteness are not abnormal. They are the great driving force of mankind, the real motivation in life.

But what if the feelings of inferiority are too strong? What if instead of motivating us to better things, these feelings cause unhappiness, discouragement, frustration, a sense of inadequacy, or feelings of worthlessness?

Causes of inferiority feelings

Psychologists and psychiatrists have had a gala day in trying to discover why so many people feel inferior!

We must first recognize that some of us feel inferior because in many respects we *are* inferior. When it comes to preparing a salad, broiling a steak, or baking a cake, I know that I am inferior to my wife. Most of us recognize we have many inferiorities that bother us very little, if at all.

But what if there is an area in which we want to do well and can't? What about the teenager who wants to get on the school basketball team, but isn't good enough? What about the college senior who wants to go to medical school, but whose grades are too low? What about the career girl who wants to get married but fears that she is not attractive? People often have strong feelings of inferiority because they are not successful in areas where they want very much to succeed. I once counseled with a man in his early twenties with many failures behind him. Everything he did seemed to turn out wrong; he had come to feel very inferior and inadequate. And, as a matter of fact, there are many indications that he felt inferior because he really *was*.

Other people feel inferior because they *think* they are inferior, even though they might not be. Most of us have met individuals who are really very capable (perhaps even outstanding) in their accomplishments, but who don't believe it. We may know people who have great potential but who don't think they can succeed.

There are several reasons why these capable people get the idea that they are inferior and inadequate. In the first place, many come to think of themselves as being inferior because they have been belittled by others. If parents, teachers or spouses repeat enough times that a person is no good, stupid, and unlikely to amount to anything - he will soon believe it.

At the opposite extreme are those people who think they are inferior because they have been pushed beyond their capacities by well-meaning but insensitive parents or other adults. When standards are set unrealistically high, failure and feelings of inferiority become inevitable. Some parents perpetually demand more than a child can produce. Eventually the youngster concludes, "I can never satisfy them," so he gives up in frustration.

Closely related to this is a third reason why people think they are inferior: frequent failure. Some very capable people who have understanding and encouraging parents, who are not pushed beyond their capabilities, still have inferiority problems. Why? Because of various circumstances these people experience frequent failure, and they convince themselves they are no good. The person who fails because of frequent illness or "bad breaks" is an example.

Sin in our lives is a fourth reason for thinking we are inferior, and a very common cause of inferiority in Christians. When a person sins, or engages in some action which goes against his conscience, there are often feelings of guilt, self-condemnation, and inferiority. Forgetting the loving and merciful Savior who forgives and forgets our sins, this person remains in his guilt. He concludes that he is a worthless person and that something is wrong with his spiritual life because he is continually tempted and so often yields.

Over-protection can also cause people to feel inferior. By dominating, smothering and fluttering over children, parents sometimes prevent their offspring from making any mistakes. Children therefore are ill-prepared for life and when they reach adulthood they experience many failures and accompanying feelings of inferiority.

Of course many people rise above the adverse circumstances of life and feel no inferiority in spite of their being belittled, pushed, unsuccessful, sinful, part of a rejected group or overprotected. It all depends on how we react to circumstances and how we handle our failures. For some, failure is a spur to greater effort and success, but for many others these problems of life lead to increased feelings of inadequacy and inferiority.

To this point we have assumed inferiority feelings are something unpleasant, but it seems some people actually enjoy feeling inferior. Certainly there are benefits to be gained from convincing ourselves and others that we are inadequate in some way. When we claim to be inferior, other people can feel sorry for us, giving us extra privileges and extra attention. And the person who belittles himself has another advantage: he never has to face the pain of attempting something and discovering that he really is a failure. A common example are students who frequently belittle themselves in front of teachers or classmates. "I just can't do math," a young girl might complain. This gets sympathy from her parents (and sometimes from a teacher or classmates) and it becomes an acceptable excuse to avoid taking a math course; it also provides a convenient excuse in case the student does poorly in the course.

The problem with convincing others that we are inferior is that before long we end up convincing ourselves. If we try to persuade other people that we cannot do mathematics, before long we believe it ourselves, and we actually do poorly in the course even though we may have high ability and high scores in mathematical aptitude tests (Figure below).

And if we succeed in convincing ourselves that we are inferior, in order to be consistent with our own convictions we act in an inferior way. Notice in the diagram that once we put in an inferior performance, this "proves" to ourselves and to others that we are indeed inferior.

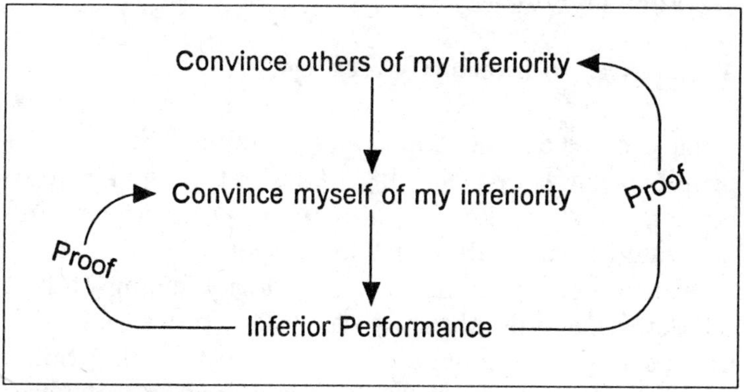

The Vicious Circle of Inferiority. The person who tries to convince others of his inferiority eventually convinces himself. Then, in order to be consistent with his belief he acts in an inferior way. This, in turn, proves to the individual and others that he really is inferior.

A person can get on to the cycle at any point and when he moves in the direction of the arrows, his feelings of inferiority increase and his performance gets worse.

Before leaving this we should note that we rarely belittle *everything* about ourselves. Instead the tendency is to downgrade ourselves in the areas we most want to succeed. In the words of one psychiatrist, "The capacities that are belittled are usually the ones in which the individual desires most ardently to excel . . . This connection is so usual that one may guess from the focus of the self-belittling tendency where the greatest ambitions lie."[3] The person who makes an issue of his intellectual inferiority often wants to succeed in that very area. The musician who makes an issue of his musical inferiority or the housewife who complains about her inability to cook are often most anxious about succeeding in those areas most frequently mentioned.

Alternatives to inferiority feelings

What can we do about inferiority feelings? For a lot of people the answer is, "Nothing." They go through life browbeaten, unhappy, convinced of their worthlessness, and frustrated because they feel so inferior.

Certain others attack their inferiority feelings, but in self-defeating and unhealthy ways. Many times we do this unconsciously, without realizing what we are doing. Some people, for example, hide their insecurities and never acknowledge that they feel inferior. Sometimes such people display a loud bombastic appearance of great self-confidence. To the world they look very self-assured but this is really a front which hides their insecurities and feelings of incompetence. For others, hidden feelings of inferiority come out in the form of physical problems like ulcers, asthma or migraine headaches. When this happens the illness is often used as a convenient excuse for inactivity and continued feelings of inferiority. Another self-defeating attitude is to wallow in one's inferiorities and to talk about them whenever the opportunity arises. By their actions, and sometimes by their words, these people make a sympathy play. "Poor little me," they complain, "look how tough life is for me and how inferior I am." Such people almost take pride in their inferiorities and sometimes they develop a "my-inferiorities-are-better-than-your-inferiorities" attitude. These are often the people who unconsciously set their goals so high that failure and continued feelings of inferiority are assured.

Another self-defeating reaction is to criticize and to knock down everyone else so that (in our own minds) we are the "top-dog." This is what the Pharisees did in Jesus' day (Matthew 23). They criticized everybody and walked around in smug superiority. The person who is highly critical is also frequently insecure and concerned about his inferiorities.

Hiding one's inferiorities, wallowing in them, or becoming highly critical of others may all seem like foolish ways for dealing with feelings of inferiority, but the people who adopt these techniques often are unwilling to change. They go through life always feeling inferior but persisting in those self-defeating activities which maintain the status quo and prevent the person from living a more pleasant and satisfying life.

Happily, however, people who feel so inferior as to be defeated need not go on through life with those feelings. There are effective ways we can handle our inadequacies. To begin, it is important to recognize that people can feel inferior both in terms of their worth and in terms of their ability. These should not be confused. In terms of *worth* all men are equal. A person's race, wealth, sex, status and responsibilities have nothing to do with how he is seen by God. In God's sight all men are of equal worth. This does not imply, however, that all men have equal *ability*. Because of special capacities, intellectual endowment, experiences and past opportunities, people differ in their accomplishments and capabilities. In terms of abilities and gifts, therefore, all men are not created equal.

The Apostle Paul recognized this and wrote that people

have different gifts and different responsibilities. When he looked at himself, Paul admitted that he wasn't as intelligent as some other men, that he didn't speak in lofty words of wisdom, that he had a tendency to be nervous and that he was physically unattractive. But Paul also recognized that he was a good writer, that he was being used of God and that he was a faithful soldier of Jesus Christ. You will note Paul didn't hide his weaknesses, he didn't wallow in them and he didn't boast of his strengths in an attempt to be superior to everyone else. And he didn't criticize or knock everyone else down. Instead he said, in essence, "I am moving out to serve Christ in the best that I can, recognizing that I have both strengths and weaknesses." *A willingness to take a realistic self-appraisal,* therefore, *is the first step* in dealing with our inferiorities.

The second healthy approach to this problem is somewhat similar: *we can change our self-image.* As we grow into adulthood, all people develop a number of opinions, attitudes and feelings about themselves. These opinions, which psychologists lump together and call self-opinions, self-concepts or self-image, develop as a result of our experiences with other people and with objects. A basketball player may recognize that he is a good athlete because of his past experience in handling the ball and because of the acclaim given by the fans. If he is well liked by the girls, but has difficulty in chemistry, he decides that he is a good athlete and a good date, but a poor student. These conclusions become part of his self-image. Since we all have different abilities, past experiences, and physical skills, we all differ in our self-concepts.

Behavior largely depends on our self-concept or to say it more simply, how we act depends on what we think of ourselves and how we see ourselves.

But what if we haven't had such experiences? Can we

train ourselves to think positively? Norman Vincent Peale thought so and wrote a book entitled *The Power of Positive Thinking* that sold millions of copies. Dale Carnegie thought so and influenced millions of people with his two books that encouraged people to change their self-image: *How to Win Friends and Influence People* and *Stop Worrying and Start Living*. Psychologists tend to be skeptical of self-help books like these, perhaps because we are jealous of their popularity. But even the stuffiest of psychological writers will recognize that self-image is important and can be changed. It is possible to think of yourself differently and this in turn can influence your actions. A more positive self-image, therefore, works against feelings of inferiority.

A third healthy way in which we can overcome feelings of inferiority *is to attack our feelings head-on and attempt to change our behavior.* If we are Number Two, we can always try harder to be Number One. Still, a competitive struggle to be the man at the top is not always desirable, nor is it satisfying. Probably most of us would agree with Adler that there is a better way to change our behavior, a more satisfying solution to the problem of inferiority. This does not come from competition with other men. It comes instead as a man strives with himself to outdo his own past performances. Everyone has heard of Winston Churchill's unimpressive career as a student, but Churchill overcame his scholastic difficulties and rose to become one of the greatest statesmen and writers in British history. Consider Franklin D. Roosevelt who had polio but overcame this to become President. Teddy Roosevelt had been a weakling in his youth and became a physically stalwart man. These men knew their strengths and weaknesses and they accepted them; but then they went on to develop their strengths and to overcome their weaknesses.

Attempting to improve on our own past behavior can, therefore, be an effective way of countering feelings of inferiority.

IMPLICATIONS FOR CHRISTIANS

Followers of Christ are likely to feel a little uncomfortable about the suggestion that we should think of ourselves more positively, that we should strive to outdo ourselves, or that we should recognize our good characteristics and attempt to improve them. Somehow this seems unchristian and wrong for people who often sing of ". . . such a worm as I."

I once counseled with a fine young lady who felt that it was Christian to be inferior. She found numerous Bible verses to support the position that to be humble meant that a Christian should be inferior and a failure. This student made the mistaken assumption that humility and inferiority are the same thing, but they are not. Inferiority refers to a persistent dwelling on one's undesirable actions and characteristics; humility implies that we can accept our strong points and that we realize both our nothingness before God, and the fact that God has given all of us certain gifts, abilities and responsibilities. According to the Bible, all men are sinners; all are nothing when contrasted with the glory and greatness of God (Romans 3:23). But God loves us. He recognizes that we are helpless and He sent His Son to die for us. When an individual acknowledges his sinful status and asks God to control his life, Christ transforms that person. The believer becomes a new creature, a child of God, and a joint heir with Christ of God's blessings (2 Corinthians 5:17). How can one feel inferior, then, when he is the object of

God's love and concern, when he has been redeemed by the Son of God, and when he is given such attention by the Creator of the universe? The Christian shouldn't bemoan his inferiority. On the contrary, he should rejoice because of his new position in Christ's family. It is true that we didn't deserve to be God's children. It is true that eternal life comes as a gift and not as a payment for our good works (Ephesians 2:8, 9). But it is also true that we have been elevated to a position of close friendship with the God of the universe. This is a reason for rejoicing!

Too often we forget that. We look at the world around us with its values and its scorn of Christianity and we assume that our religion really does attract inferior people. Before long we begin to think that we are inferior. We belittle ourselves and others, or we set impossible standards for ourselves. We over-protect ourselves by withdrawing from the world into secure little cloisters. After a while we begin to feel safe and to enjoy our withdrawn state. We learn to love our self-centered worship, we enjoy wallowing in our assumed inferiorities and we criticize others because they are not as spiritual or humble as we are.

This kind of thinking needs to be changed. We must stop apologizing for our devotion to and dependence on a living God. It is time that we honestly acknowledge that while we are all sinners, we are valuable creatures because God created us, loves us and sent His Son to redeem us. If we have invited Christ into our lives we are new creatures set apart to serve the living God. We don't all have the same gifts or abilities and we don't all have the same responsibilities. God doesn't call everyone to be a teacher or a deacon or a foreign missionary, but we do all have the same call to serve with whatever we have to give. According to the Bible every part of the body of Christ is necessary and important (1 Corinthians 12:14-28). Periodically, therefore, we must pause to acknowledge these facts, to confess our inferiorities to Christ, and to commit our lives wholly to Him. Then both of our self-image and our behavior will change.

Do you feel inferior? To some extent this isn't bad. It may mean that you honestly recognize your weaknesses as well as your strengths. It may mean that you realize your place in God's universe. It could even spur you on to do better. But let's keep the Scriptures in perspective. Wallowing in our inferiorities, taking pride in having admitted them, is sinful. It involves a failure to accept the fact that God has actually changed us and given us abilities that can be used for His service. The writer of the Book of James gives good advice: humble yourselves in the sight of the Lord, but then remember that "Christ shall lift you up" (James 4:10). Let us not take such pleasure in our inferiorities that we refuse to be lifted up, that we refuse to be used or that we refuse to think as God intended his people to think.

8

Discouragement

Discouragement is as old as man himself. If we look into the Bible, for example, we discover that there were many times in the ancient past when people showed discouragement. The Old Testament records one situation when the children of Israel became "much discouraged" in the midst of their wilderness wanderings (Numbers 20:14-21). The people had been in the wilderness for a long time and probably were tired. Miriam, Moses' sister, had died recently and the people had experienced a long drought. They were clearly in a complaining mood as they arrived at the borders of the country called Edom. Edom was shaped somewhat like the letter "U" and to get past this country the children of Israel had two alternatives. They could either go directly across the country from one side to the other or they could walk a long detour around. The King of Edom came out with a mighty army and made it very clear what would happen if the Israelites dared to step one foot onto Edomite territory. Faced with the prospect of going the long way around Edom, the Israelites became even more discouraged.

Today still – we see that there are many people in the

world - including committed Christians - who are very unhappy and discouraged. So common is the problem we could say that the person who never gets discouraged is unusual and in many respects abnormal.

The causes of discouragement

1 One of the most common reasons behind discouragement is **frustration over our inability to accomplish some task.** When a person gets frustrated because he can't succeed at doing something he often gets discouraged at the same time. Sometimes this frustration and discouragement come because the task is too long or too time-consuming.

Students frequently get discouraged when they are a long way from completing their course of study. When the student arrives at college, he comes with an enthusiasm which often continues through the first year. When the novelty and excitement wear off and the student comes back for his second year of study, he recognizes that the road ahead is very long, and he gets frustrated and discouraged. In the USA, among students, suicide is now the second most frequent cause of death.

People also get frustrated and then discouraged when a task is too difficult. Related to this is the frustration and discouragement which come because a project just doesn't seem to succeed. Moses, Joshua, Elijah, Job and David were each discouraged because things didn't go the way they had hoped. Jeremiah preached his heart out but nobody responded (except with occasional laughter) and he became a very discouraged "weeping prophet." People today get discouraged when they aren't successful in molding children, winning a contest or an election as they had hoped, getting a job or an award of some kind, or being given a good grade on a test. Sometimes we even set up goals that we cannot possibly reach and then feel discouraged because of our lack of anticipated success.

2 A second major cause of discouragement is **the behavior of others.** The Scriptures instruct fathers not to provoke their children lest these little ones become discouraged (Colossians 3:21). The word "provoke" means to irritate or to be too exacting and sometimes we get discouraged because people provoke us. They put impossibly high demands on us (or at least we think their demands are too high) or they are highly critical of something we have done or failed to do. Because of these actions or criticisms from others, we get discouraged.

3 A third major cause of discouragement is **separation from people we love and respect.** Everyone knows the sadness and discouragement that are usually present when a loved one has died. Terminally ill patients and their families get discouraged not only because of the frustration of a long disease but also because of their dread of the coming separation.[1] "I won't be with them anymore," the patient thinks - and his relatives prepare for a new kind of life without the loved one. Little children who have no real time sense, show despair and discouragement when they are hospitalized.[2] Older people are sad and feel a sense of loss when their children go away to school, when a couple goes to the mission field, or whenever there is some other kind of temporary separation. Some sickness reflects discouragement: a grief reaction brought on by separation.

4 Some writers have suggested that a **lack of purpose in life** can also cause discouragement. Philosophers talk about existential despair, a deep discouragement which comes because men have no direction and no apparent meaning in life. This lack of purpose may explain the discouragement of drifting college students, of housewives whose lives seem to consist primarily of doing dishes and changing diapers, or people in their 40's and 50's who are disappointed because they have not accomplished more in life but who see little hope for change.

5 We must recognize that sometimes the primary cause of discouragement is **physical**. Women who have recently had a baby or who are going through the menopause may be prone to discouragement, usually because of hormone imbalance. And we know that both men and women when tired, hungry, "out of shape," or not feeling well, have a lowered ability to resist discouragement.

6 All of this does not hide the fact, however, that the causes of discouragement are often **spiritual**. In writing to the Corinthian church, the Apostle Paul indicated that he had experienced discouragement and he seemed to blame this on the devices of Satan (2 Corinthians 2:1-11). To get people depressed must surely be a tactic of the Devil who wants to see people, especially Christian people, ineffective, unproductive, and hindered in their work (1 Thessalonians 2:18). There is also the possibility, however, that some of our discouragement comes from God. He too may hinder our earthly ambitions and this could lead to discouragement, especially when we fail to grasp the wisdom of God's divine plan for our lives.

CHARACTERISTICS OF DISCOURAGEMENT

How do discouraged people act? Most obvious are feelings of sadness, unhappiness, frustration and disappointment. There may be tears and crying, accompanied sometimes by worry, anxiety about the future, or a desire to be alone and unbothered by others. Sometimes the person feels guilty and angry with himself, especially if he knows that the discouraging situation was his own fault.

Discouraged persons often find fault and criticize strangers, their fellow workers, their neighbors, other Christians, their families and sometimes even God. We see the tendency of discouraged people to bemoan their fate and wallow in their problems. Then there is apathy, which leads to slowing down and perhaps stopping our normal activities.

Even people whose discouragement is mild lose the motivation and enthusiasm to keep pushing on with their activities. Sometimes these people get careless in their grooming. They may stop eating. And they don't bother to spend time in prayer or Bible study.

These symptoms and the discouragement which they reflect are very common. Almost everyone gets discouraged at times and in mild form we show many of the above characteristics. Most of us, however, can rise above our troubles sooner or later, but there are some who can't recover quite that easily. They sink into deep despair, sometimes even when the problem is relatively minor or when there are hopeful signs of improvement. Such deeply depressed people are perpetually unhappy, withdrawn socially, inactive, and plagued with feelings of hopelessness, helplessness, and deep despondency. Often there is intense anxiety, concern over physical aches and pains, and a tendency to blame one's self for the trials of life. This intense type of discouragement is beyond the scope of this book. It is usually dealt with by a competent psychiatrist, psychologist, or other mental health professional.

Dealing with discouragement

There are at least six healthy ways to deal with discouragement.

1 First, we can **recognize and accept the fact that all of us get discouraged at times.** This is part of being human.

Remember that God, who controls the universe and causes or permits discouraging situations to arise, knows what He is doing and why. But we cannot comprehend God's plan with our small brains and from our limited perspective. Remember Job? God and Satan talked together about Job's troubles (Job 1:1-12; 2:1-6), but, according to the Bible, Job never knew why he experienced his problems.

Still, in His mercy God has given us some hints as to why discouragement and other problems come into our lives. Sometimes difficulties are to bring glory to God. This is why Lazarus was allowed to die (John 11:4). Sometimes the problems bring spiritual growth, greater patience, and more humility on the part of the sufferer or people who knew him (John 11:15; 1 Peter 1:6-7). At times God chastises us as an expression of His love (Hebrews 12:6). More often, however, we simply cannot understand why God acts the way He does or why problems enter our lives. Instead we must accept the difficult conclusion that a discouraging situation is with us for reasons we cannot understand (Romans 11:33).

2 A second healthy reaction to discouragement **is trust – a renewed dependence on God** (Psalm 42:5). Like Job, in the midst of his trials and discouragements, we must learn to say, "Though He slay me, yet will I trust in Him" (Job 13:15). This isn't very easy. Many people trust God can save us eternally, but they do not trust He will be with us on earth, even though He has promised to do so (Jude 24; 2 Thessalonians 3:3; Matthew 28:20).

3 This brings us to a third healthy reaction to discouragement – **meaningful activity**. The discouraged person should remain active, should resist the temptation to sit around in despair and self-pity. The best kind of activity is that which is directed towards improving our undesirable situation and making things different.

4 Fourth, to overcome discouragement **we need to keep perspective**. When we experience an emotion like discouragement it is often easy to look for the bad in the situation and never to see the good. Here is one place where a concerned Christian friend can help as the discouraged person talks over the problem, expresses his feelings, gets a more realistic evaluation of the situation, and considers some practical ways of improvement. We may have to change our behavior in some way or attempt to see the situation as others see it.

5 Closely related to this is a fifth suggestion – trying to **uncover the causes of the discouragement**. Certainly it isn't always easy to understand the causes of one's feeling. Sometimes we need a friend or counselor to help us see the source of our unhappiness.

6 Finally, we need to **be alert to our physical condition.** Plenty of sleep, periodic exercise, and a balanced diet

can all help us meet existing discouragements and be less overwhelmed by problems in the future.

Implications for Christians

We have a cause for happiness but we must never get the idea that it is unchristian or unspiritual for people to be unhappy at times. Periodic discouragement is a part of life and although believers can always be glad for their relationship with Christ and for their awareness of His sovereignty, there is nothing in the Bible to imply that we should always be grinning with happiness and bubbling over with exuberance. On the contrary, there are times when a Christian should weep.

Dr. John R.W. Stott of All Souls Church in London made a systematic study of the Bible and identified several times when weeping is appropriate.[3] Stott has distinguished between "tears of nature and tears of grace."

The first of these, tears of nature, come because we are human. These are tears that flow in response to the trials of life, when we are parting, when we are grieving, or when others are having problems (1 Peter 1:6; 2 Timothy 1:4; Acts 20:37; John 11:35; Romans 12:15). In such situations the Christian can be aware of God's presence and God's control but he might also weep. We do not sorrow like those who have no hope (1 Thessalonians 4:13), but there is nothing wrong in sadness and crying. Jesus wept at a funeral. Indeed, it is quite natural and part of our humanity.

The second type of tears, the tears of grace, are shed because we are believers. These tears are rare among Christians today but were present in Bible times. This includes tears over our own sin (Ezra 10:1; Psalm 119:136; Philippians 3:18), and weeping over the lost condition or sin of others. Jesus shed tears when He wept over Jerusalem (Luke 19:41).

Dr. Stott concludes his perceptive article with these words:

> The fundamental error underlying our modern tearlessness is a misunderstanding of God's plan of salvation, a false assumption that His saving work is finished, that its benefits may be enjoyed completely, and that there is no need for any more sickness, suffering, or sin, which are the causes of sorrow.
>
> This is just not true. . . . The fruits of this salvation have not yet been fully garnered. And they will not be, and cannot be, until the end comes when Christ returns in power and glory. The ravages of the Fall have not yet been eradicated either in the world or in Christian people. We have a fallen nature, an ingrained corruption, over which to weep. We still live in a fallen world, full of sorrow, full of suffering and sin . . .
>
> . . . The eyes that do not weep are blind eyes – eyes closed to the facts of sin and of suffering in ourselves and in the rest of humanity. . . .[4]

A time is coming when there will be no more crying, suffering or despair; until then, however, let us recognize that problems and discouragement will be part of our lives even when we are committed Christians. Let us realize that the Holy Spirit will comfort and guide in times of discouragement, and then let us rejoice – in the midst of our life on earth – as we recognize the sovereignty of God, His guidance in the present, and His promise for the future.

9

Homosexuality*

CONSIDERING "SEXUAL DEVIATIONS"

There are large individual differences in homosexual behavior. Some people are exclusively homosexual while others are sexually attracted to both sexes. Some are basically heterosexual but engage in homosexual acts when in prison, the military, boarding schools, or other situations when the opposite sex is not around. For some people, their attraction to the same sex is so well-hidden that it is not recognized even by themselves. Others recognize that they have homosexual tendencies but are able to keep this a secret. Still others are overt homosexuals who freely engage in sexual relations with members of the same sex, "marry" their homosexual partners, and worship together in "homosexual churches."

There are a number of misconceptions about homosexuality that should be discarded. For example, while many of these people are self-centered, immature, lonely and unhappy (not really "gay"), this does not mean that

* From *Fractured Personalities* by Gary Collins, © 1972, Creation House.

they are mentally ill. On the contrary, most homosexuals, like most heterosexuals, show no evidence of serious emotional disturbances.[1] Furthermore, homosexuals are not necessarily distinguishable by their physique or actions. While some male homosexuals are of slight build and effeminate in their mannerisms, many others are athletic, virile-looking men who give no hint of femininity. Also, there is no evidence to support the popular idea that homosexuals are especially creative. These people often engage in creative work, such as acting, hairdressing or interior decorating, but they are no more creative, productive or intelligent than nonhomosexuals.[2] Finally, *it should not be assumed that homosexuality is organically caused*. While there is still disagreement on this, most experts agree that *homosexuality is an acquired condition* wherein a person learns to fear and avoid the opposite sex, often because of his past experiences or upbringing. Of course the reasons for homosexuality are complex, and no one explanation can cover all cases.[3]

Causes, treatment and prevention of deviations

Sex deviates show a multitude of symptoms, their behavior may have any number of causes, and they can be treated with a variety of techniques. Studies of sexually maladjusted people frequently reveal one or more of the following: lack of opportunity to engage in normal sex behavior, isolation in childhood, unusual experiences in childhood or adolescence in which deviant sexuality is learned, fear of the opposite sex, fear of being hurt if one engages in normal sex, lack of opportunity to learn appropriate sex roles (e.g., in homes where there is no father, boys have difficulty learning how to act like a male), fear of adult responsibilities, sexual ignorance, and belief that normal sexual behavior is dirty and sinful.[4]

Medical treatment tends to be ineffective. Instead, it appears that psychotherapy and other kinds of psychological treatment are the most successful. But deviates often do not want to change. Their way of getting sexual satisfaction is pleasant and, inspite of social criticism, there is frequently a desire to persist in the deviation.

It is clear then that prevention is extremely important. Accurate sex education, preparation for healthy marital relationships, the alleviation of abnormal family situations, and guidance as the person grows to maturity, can all be important.[5] In each of these preventive measures, the church can play a role.

Sexual deviation and the church

Society, in general, treats the sexually deviate person with great scorn, and many church people prefer to think that it is impossible to be a Christian and a sexual deviate. When deviation is discovered, there are shocked disbelief and immediate efforts to purge the congregation and community of such people. The deviate, in turn, comes to view himself as being dirty, "queer," unwanted, and something less than human.[6]

The Bible specifically condemns many of the sexual perversions. In the Old Testament law, the acts of incest, extramarital relations, homosexuality and sexual experiences with animals are all mentioned by name, described as sin, and specifically prohibited (Leviticus 18:6-18, 20, 22-24, 30). The New Testament speaks against prostitution, fornication (premarital sex), adultery (extramarital sex), and homosexuality (Hebrews 13:4; 1 Corinthians 7:1-2; 1 Thessalonians 4:3; Romans 1:21-27). When the

Bible talks of sex, it is referring to the union of a man and a woman who love each other and are "one flesh" in marriage (Hebrews 13:4; Ephesians 5:28-31; Matthew 19:5-6). To fit perversions into the biblical view of sex,

> "Is impossible at every point. The sex act in marriage is the ultimate expression of love. The sex act performed apart from marriage falls short of this ultimate expression and leaves much to be desired. Often, if not always, it leaves both persons with a sense of guilt and lack of fulfillment. This is true of loveless marriage, of masturbation, and of homosexual activity."[7]

Faced with the reality of widespread sexual abuse and perversion, church leaders and other Christians have the following responsibilities:

Acceptance of the sexually deviate The woman taken in adultery (John 8) and the woman at the well (John 4) had both been participating in sexually deviant behavior. Jesus did not approve of their sinful actions, but He did accept them as people in need.

We must also accept them for what they are - individuals whom Christ loves, and people who need a special way to experience the power and grace of God. Although He was criticized for doing so, Jesus spent time with publicans and sinners since these were the people whom He came to redeem. In like manner, we who are followers of Christ cannot cast off the sexual deviate as a hopeless untouchable.

Counseling Sex deviates can profit from a frank discussion of their sexual problems, but counseling with these people is a very difficult task, especially if the counselor has little formal training or understanding of the problem. Exhorting the deviate to "change his ways" or to bury his problem under activities is usually ineffective,[8] and it may be more efficient to encourage the person to seek the help of a professional counselor.

Education Church members should be taught both about deviations and about the biblical standards for mature sexual expression. An understanding of these facts is important if we are to prevent deviation and help those who are having sexual problems.

10

Mental Health and Prevention of Abnormality

Mental health is too large a concept to be defined in a few words. Instead, it is more realistic to see what mental health is *not* and then to list some of the characteristics that indicate good *mental health*. According to a group of professional counselors, mental health is *not*

1 Adjustment under all circumstances. There are many circumstances to which man should not adjust, otherwise there would be no progress.

2 Freedom from anxiety and tensions. Anxiety and tension are often prerequisites and accompaniments of creativity and self-preservation . . .

3 Freedom from dissatisfaction. . . .

4 Conformity. One criterion of maturity is the ability to stand apart from the crowd when conditions indicate. . . .

5 Constant happiness. In this imperfect world, a sensitive, mature person often experiences unhappiness.

6 A lessening of accomplishment and creativity. Mental health is characterized by the ability of the individual to use his powers ever more fully.

7 The absence of personal idiosyncrasies. Many such idiosyncrasies which do not interfere with function enrich the life of the individual and those who come in contact with him.

8 The undermining of authority. Mental health is characterized by the increased ability of the individual to use and respect realistic authority while deprecating the use of authority as an oppressive force. . . .

9 Opposition to religious values. Mental health facilitates and complements the aims of religion inasmuch as it fosters the highest spiritual and social values.[1]

There is no sharp line between mental health and mental illness, between being normal and abnormal. Most people are some place in between, and in all probability vascillate back and forth on the scale of mental health as problems and crises come into their lives.

Some characteristics of good mental health

The mentally healthy person will probably show many of these more important characteristics of mental health:

Social and emotional competence Mentally healthy persons generally behave in ways which are acceptable to the majority of people in the society. Each acts in accordance with the social roles typical for one of his age, sex, education, marital status and occupation. He respects the rights and needs of others, accepts responsibility for his own actions, tries to understand and appreciate the motives of others, and helps those in need. He is not immobilized by fear, anger, love or anxiety, but neither does he hide these and other emotions, pretending they do not exist.

Satisfying interpersonal relations According to Erich Fromm, the famous psychoanalyst, man wants to be unique, but he also needs to be related to other people in bonds of mutual care, responsibility, respect and understanding.[2] The normal person has both superficial social contacts and intimate, deeply involved relationships with one or a few confidants.

Self-examination and insight More than 2,000 years ago Socrates said that "the unexamined life is not worth living." Jesus instructed His followers to look at the faults in their own lives before criticizing others (Matthew 7:1-5). When He instituted the Lord's Supper, Jesus told each one to "examine himself" before partaking of the elements (1 Corinthians 11:27-30).

If we honestly look at ourselves we should get some insight into our behavior and some appreciation for both our strengths and weaknesses. Of course, it is difficult to be objective in our self-examination and we should realize that no one ever achieves complete self-insight. But we will get along better if we have at least some self-understanding. It also helps if we have a sense of humor. Life is serious, but nevertheless the normal individual is able to get things in perspective and occasionally to laugh at himself and his circumstances.

Self-acceptance and self-confidence Self-examination often reveals things about ourselves that we don't want to see, and can lead to pessimism, self-pity, self-rejection, and a loss of self-confidence. But the mentally healthy individual is not overwhelmed by his own weaknesses. He can pray, "God grant me the serenity to accept the things I cannot change, the courage to change the things I can, and the wisdom to know the difference." Recognizing his strong points along with the weak, he accepts himself for what he is, improves where he can, sets realistic aspirations, and works to build his self-confidence.

Realistic approach to problems It is not healthy to evade problems, hide from them, or try to solve them through excessive worry, complaining, or procrastination.[3] Even though it may be painful, the healthy person faces his problems realistically and tries to arrive at successful solutions. To some extent this involves being organized, so that the individual is not overwhelmed by his problems and responsibilities but can handle them one at a time.

Freedom from internal conflict, intense feelings of insecurity, and paralyzing anxiety The mentally healthy person cannot be immobilized by such internal tension and turmoil.

Satisfying philosophy of life To be mentally healthy is to have some meaning to life and some purpose for living. The healthy person also holds values and moral principles which guide his behavior and influence his thinking.

The Bible contains many guidelines for satisfying life. In Philippians 2, for example, we are admonished to think like Christ (v. 5) who was obedient and humble (v. 8). We are able to do things without grumbling (v. 14) and to shine as examples of godly behavior living "in a world of corrupt and sinful people" (v. 15). But the really satisfying life comes only when we "openly proclaim that Jesus Christ is Lord" (v. 11) and invite Him to control our lives so that He will help us "want to obey Him, and . . . do what He wants" (v. 13, *LB*). This is old theology - some would call it old-fashioned - but it is good theology, and a basic requirement for real mental health.

Love A specific description of love is given in 1 Corinthians 13:4-8:

> "Love is patient and kind; love is not jealous or boastful; it is not arrogant or rude. Love does not insist on its own way; it is not irritable or resentful; it does not rejoice at wrong, but rejoices in the right. Love bears all things, believes all things, hopes all things, endures all things. Love never ends."

Complete normality is a rare state possessed only by people who are at peace with society, with themselves, and with God. The characteristics listed above are consistent with this threefold definition of mental health.

Prevention of abnormal behavior

There are two common approaches to the prevention of abnormal behavior. We can work to prevent the development of new disorders (primary prevention), or we can try to spot mild disorders and prevent them from becoming more serious or prolonged (secondary prevention).

Primary prevention

If we hope to prevent abnormal behavior from developing, we must reduce or eliminate early experience that could be psychologically harmful, and we must teach people how to handle stresses of life. In preventing abnormality it is important to be alert to the biological, psychological, social and spiritual spheres of life.

Biological prevention Good physical health and good mental health do not always go together, but they do frequently. If a person takes care of his physical needs, has a balanced diet, takes time for exercise and relaxation, avoids overindulgence in food, drugs or alcohol, and gets sufficient sleep, he will be better able to handle life's stresses.

Psychological prevention Education is of crucial importance in preventing psychological disorders. Parents must learn how to live in harmony with each other and to provide a home where there is a minimum of tension, neglect of children, overpermissiveness or overprotection. Children must be taught discipline and responsibility, must acquire the roles and social expectations of their society, must learn how to handle the stresses of life, and must be guided as they prepare for the future.

Spiritual prevention By developing clear-cut moral standards, finding an enduring faith, and formulating a unifying philosophy of life, people are immunizing themselves against psychological collapse. Primarily the home and the church are responsible for instilling these moral standards, but many parents have ignored their duty, concluding that "children should decide what they believe when they get older."

Secondary prevention

Once an emotional disorder has begun, three things can be done to stop it before it blossoms into a more serious abnormality.

We must detect developing problems. This is the responsibility of everyone in the community: teachers, doctors, employers, pastors, Sunday School teachers, etc. Of all these people, the church leader probably is in the best position for locating people with developing problems. He sees members of the congregation from week to week, knows their families, and can observe them in a variety of settings, including the church, home, and social gatherings. It is a good idea to watch for high-risk groups such as children from broken homes, the grief-stricken, adolescents, the elderly, the physically ill, and the socially deprived, for all these have a higher than average likelihood of developing disorders.[4]

Get the person to a place where he can be helped. People with developing problems are often not very motivated to get help. Their "problem" may not be bothering them much (in cases such as drinking, drug use, sex deviations or some neurotic re-actions, they may actually be enjoying their abnormal behavior) so there is little desire to take the time or effort to engage in counseling. Motivation is often improved when the person is helped to see the logical outcome of his present behavior, and his need to seek help.

Get the necessary help for stopping and hopefully eliminating the developing abnormality. The goal is not to remold the personality, but to work toward eliminating symptoms so the counselee can return to efficient functioning in his society,[5] and know how to handle recurring problems on his own.

Mental health and the church

While establishing mental health in the community is not the church's primary role, if we believe that the Christian message has relevance to the needs of contemporary man then we are responsible for bringing Christianity's resources to bear on the problems of those in our congregations and communities. There are at least ten practical ways in which church leaders can do this; all are consistent with biblical revelation and psychologically sound:*

1 Introduce men and women to Jesus Christ The Bible does not promise that Christianity is a ticket to permanent mental health. The follower of Jesus Christ must bear a cross (Matthew 16:24; Mark 8:34; 10:21; Luke 9:23) and commit himself to a costly form of discipleship. Becoming a Christian often creates problems we could otherwise avoid. Why, then, should we encourage men and women to invite Christ into their lives? One reason is that by following Christ we have a challenging purpose in life (to follow Him), and a reason for living (Matthew 16:24-25; 2 Corinthians 5:15, 17; Galatians 2:20; Philippians 1:21). In addition, belief in Christ gives us "enduring faith" and a basis for the values that many psychologists

* In preparing these ten practical suggestions, I have drawn heavily on an excellent book by Howard J. Clinebell, Jr., entitled *Mental Health Through Christian Community*.

consider to be so important. In times of crises, Jesus Christ gives support and encouragement to those who depend on Him (Matthew 11:28-30). Indeed, the whole Christian life is one of fullness (Mark 1:15; John 10:10) and this has been the experience of believers for centuries. Then, when we approach the end of life, we can face death knowing that there is eternal existence in a place prepared for those who have believed that Jesus Christ is the Son of God (John 14:1-3; 3:16).

2 **Worship** In the Old Testament, the worship of God was a central act in the life of the people. During His life on earth, Jesus reaffirmed the importance of worship both with His words (Matthew 4:10b; John 4:23) and His example (Luke 4:16). The early church worshiped together (Acts 2:47); Paul encouraged believers to pray and give thanks (1 Timothy 2:1).

Worship is more than a divine commandment however; it is an experience which encourages good mental health. For many, worship gives a feeling of oneness with others. As people sing in unison, pray together and draw near to God, they also draw closer to each other and feel less isolated. Worship that is reverent gives an awareness of God's presence, a renewed sense of trust, a feeling of superhuman strength, and opportunity to sit quietly and reflect.

Too often worship in the local church is not a meaningful experience, but is instead a dull mechanical routine. In many churches – especially evangelical Protestant churches – there is considerable chatter (which we call "fellowship") before, after and sometimes during the services. The minister shows little sense of reverence and the people are deprived of an experience which could be spiritually uplifting and psychologically invigorating.

3 Private devotions Here is another activity which was a vital part of the life of Jesus (Mark 1:35; 6:46-47; Luke 6:12) and is a must for everyone of His followers (Psalm 46; 1 Thessalonians 5:17; 1 Timothy 2:8; John 5:39). Prayer gives us strength (1 Chronicles 16:11; Luke 18:1); wisdom (Matthew 7:7; James 1:5); the ability to withstand temptations (Matthew 26:41)*; joy (John 16:24); the opportunity to express our feelings (James 5:13); and the material things that we need and that God wants us to have (1 John 5:14-15; James 4:2-3; Matthew 21:22). Quiet meditation and study of the Scriptures gives knowledge, confidence and hope (2 Timothy 2:15; John 5:39; Romans 15:4).

In this age of hyperactivity and excessive busyness, men need to be still and get to know God (Psalm 46:10). Such a quiet time is another example of behavior which is of crucial importance, both spiritually and psychologically.

4 Preaching As he seeks to proclaim the Word of God, the preacher must show how the truths of the Bible apply to men's needs and everyday problems of living. The sermon which Peter preached on the day of Pentecost (Acts 2) is a good example of speaking to people's needs, showing the relevance of Scripture, and giving opportunity for men to make a practical response to the Word of God.

5 Teaching The Sunday School hour has been called the "most wasted hour of the week." Thousands of youngsters are bored with Sunday School programs and become church drop-outs as soon as they can get out from under

* By withstanding temptation, we presumably also avoid the guilt which so often follows our yielding to temptation.

parental pressure to attend. The Christian education program is vital to the work of the church and can make a valuable contribution to mental health but, to be effective, it must be reevaluated in many local congregations.

6 **Stimulating healthy family life** Most abnormal behavior can be traced back to an unhealthy family situation. Many research studies have shown that early experience in the home is of crucial importance and even wise King Solomon recognized the importance of early training and discipline (Proverbs 22:6, 13-24).

7 **Group interaction** There are many things that a person can do alone, but being a Christian is not one of them. Jesus had a little band of twelve disciples whom He trained (Matthew 10) and sent forth as witnesses. The early church was a closely knit group that met together for study, fellowship, the "breaking of bread" and prayer (Acts 2:42). The first missionary journeys were made by teams of men.

Within the past few years churches have shown a renewed interest in small groups. Christians have discovered that there is real spiritual growth when two or more people get together to pray, study, discuss, and share their personal needs or concerns. Group experience gives a feeling of "togetherness." It shows that somebody cares, and it gives us an opportunity to be concerned about others.

8 **Service** The gospel accounts indicate that Jesus spent much time in private communion with God, and that He devoted many hours to teaching His little group of disciples. But Jesus also was highly involved in service to others. He healed the sick, ministered to the needy, and

preached from the Scriptures. Clearly He expects His followers to do likewise (Matthew 10:7-8; 28:19-20; Titus 3:8). A faith that does not lead men to do good works is a faith that is dead (James 2:17-18). The therapeutic value of service to others was discovered early by members of Alcoholics Anonymous who found that by helping others they helped themselves. The church, therefore, must encourage and mobilize the laborers. Guided by the Holy Spirit, our service will reach others and, in turn, help us both spiritually and psychologically.

9 Support in crises People who are facing crises need the help of others. The physically and mentally-ill, the discouraged, bereaved, rejected, aged, and the families of such people all need support and encouragement. As followers of Christ, who is always present when we are in need (Matthew 28:20), Christians are failing in their duty if they neglect to minister to those facing the crises of life.

10 Counseling One of the most direct contributions that the church can make to mental health is in counseling distressed people. In some communities the minister or other church leader may be the only counselor who is readily accessible; but even when other counselors are available, some people are reluctant to visit a psychologist. The minister is far less threatening and a great deal less expensive. The success of pastoral counseling depends in large measure on the church leader's training and familiarization with counseling procedures.

IV

Stress in Counseling

11

Making the Best of Stress

Originally, stress was a term used only by engineers and architects. The word referred to a force which put such pressure on an object that the object was altered in some way. Later the term stress came to be used in a much broader sense. Physical stress, emotional stress, social stress, psychological stress, and similar phrases were used to describe forces that put pressure on living organisms.

As used in this chapter, stress refers to an influence or stimulus which exerts force on a person. Broadly defined, *stress refers to any stimulation which puts pressure on a person and requires him to make difficult adjustments.* The stress may come from the external environment or from inside the individual. It may be mild or moderate or so severe that it poses a strong danger to the well-being of the person. At times it can lead to a physical or psychological collapse. If we never encountered stress, life would be simple – and also pretty dull. For most people, however, stress is a common experience. Every day we meet influences which in some way alter our behavior.

THE SOURCES OF STRESS

A situation is stressful if it hinders, makes difficult, or causes failure in some activity. Such everyday experiences as noise, distractions, competition, a lack of time, or a difficult problem can all be stressful (Korchin, 1963). Psychologists usually divide stresses into three categories: those which arise from frustrations, those resulting from conflicts, and those which stem from pressures.

Frustrations

Frustration results when our progress toward some desirable goal is blocked. **External** frustrations are obstacles in the environment. All of us have experienced rain at a picnic, a pen that runs dry in the middle of a signature, or a flat tire when we are in a hurry.

Internal frustrations refer to personal limitations within the individual. These could include physical handicaps, a low opinion of one's self, social incompetence, or a lack of desired training. Below average ability for a student who wants to be a physician or small body-build in a boy who wants to play basketball are examples of frustrations resulting from internal limitations.

Conflicts

Almost every adult has had the experience of being forced to decide between two or more mutually exclusive goals. This is a "conflict." **Approach-approach conflict** arises when the incompatible goals are equally attractive and the individual is torn between two desirable alternatives. The woman in the dress shop is in this kind of a conflict, and so is the student who wants to take anthropology and sociology but discovers they both meet at the same hour. Most people resolve this kind of conflict by choosing one goal and trying to forget the other.

Avoidance-avoidance conflict results when one is faced with two equally undesirable alternatives. When a mother says to her young daughter, "Eat your spinach or go without dessert" the child is in an avoidance-avoidance conflict. The person in pain with a toothache but who dislikes dentists is also in this kind of conflict.

Approach-avoidance conflict occurs when a goal has both desirable and undesirable features at the same time. The pastor who is called to a large church may want to serve in this greater area of influence, but may at the same time feel in doubt about his ability to handle the job. Many people experience approach-avoidance conflict as they contemplate marriage. There is a desire for the warm and loving relationship, but a fear that marriage might interfere with one's freedom, career aspirations or travel plans.

This is perhaps the most common type of conflict. It leads to great vascillation and indecision. The attractive features of the situation draw us to it, but the unattractive ones bounce us back (Arkoff, 1968).

In everyday living, few conflicts fit precisely into one of these three categories: the decisions of life are usually more complex. The pastor who is called to the large church, for example, may really be facing multiple conflicts. There may be both desirable and undesirable features connected with (a) staying in his present position (b) moving to a larger church or, perhaps (c) leaving the pastorate altogether and teaching in a seminary.

Pressures

Sometimes people experience demands that push them toward a certain type of behavior. These demands are usually termed "pressures."

External pressures come from other people or from the situation in which we are living. Parents pressure their children to get higher grades, teachers give assignments and deadlines which put pressure on their students, and religious leaders sometimes pressure their congregation to "make decisions for Christ." Probably everyone has heard of the "high pressure salesman" who tries to push prospective customers into making a purchase. Sometimes the pressure comes from a number of less specific sources. The young mother who struggles to maintain a home and keep the kids happy, and the business executive who must make many important decisions, are examples of persons who feel pressure from the environment.

Internal pressures are usually related to our ambitions or self-image. The student who feels he must get all A's, the soldier who wants to be a hero, the musician who wants to have a perfect concert, or the author who feels pushed to write a novel of highest quality, are influenced by internal pressures - all of which have been learned during the course of one's lifetime.

Frustration, conflict, and pressure often combine in a given stress situation. Let us return to the preacher who is deciding whether to move to a larger church. Since any decision has both favorable and unfavorable features, the pastor is in a multiple conflict situation. Assume, however, that in addition the other congregation is anxious for an immediate decision, and that the present congregation is urging him not to "leave such a thriving work." To these pressures might be added the frustration of wanting God's leading, but not yet knowing it. With important decisions, the stress may be great because all three sources are often present.

SEVERITY OF STRESS

All stress is not severe; some is relatively minor. According to one psychologist (Coleman, 1964), the severity of a stressful situation can be determined by considering several questions.

How long has the stress persisted? When stress lasts for a long period it tends to become more and more severe. For one night we can tolerate a loud radio playing until midnight in the next apartment. If the radio is on every night until three a.m., however, the stress (and anger) becomes more intense. Research studies have shown that even a mild stress which persists for a long time is more of a strain than an intense but brief stress (Torrance, 1965).

How important is the stress? Conflict over whether or not to marry is likely to be more important and hence more stressful than conflict over whether or not to have a second cup of coffee after dinner.

How many stresses are operating at a given time? Stresses which might be easy to handle separately, may be very difficult to handle if they all occur at once. If the dinner guests arrive, the telephone rings, the baby cries, and the timer sounds on the oven - all at the same time, - the hostess is likely to feel great stress (to put it mildly) especially if her husband has not yet arrived home from work.

Are the conflicting forces of nearly equal strength? If so, the conflict is likely to be more intense and difficult to resolve.

How does the individual look at the situation? People perceive situations differently and react in accordance with their perceptions. Two people in love may view a broken engagement in different ways. For one it may be a source of intense frustration accompanied by feelings of failure, inadequacy, and humiliation. Another may feel hurt, but also be grateful that the incompatibility became known before the marriage rather than afterwards. Obviously, the first person experiences greater stress.

How much "stress-resistance" does the individual have? "Stress tolerance" or "frustration tolerance" refers to the intensity of stress that a person can experience without undergoing a breakdown in his behavior. Apparently, there are considerable individual differences in this ability to withstand stress. What is greatly stressful for one person may be less stressful for another. Some writers have suggested that mental health involves not only functioning adequately in general but also having the ability to get along effectively while under stress (Korchin, 1963).

REACTIONS TO STRESS

The severity of stress determines, in large measure, how one will react. Mild stress leads to *improved* psychological functioning, better learning, and greater efficiency. It is not until stress becomes intense that there is a *deterioration* in one's behavior (Torrance). To put this in more practical terms, students (including those in the Sunday School) learn best if there is some pressure, but not too much. Overly permissive child rearing and overly harsh techniques can both be harmful for a child.

We may identify two broad types of stress. The first

is the brief but intense stress that comes in emergency situations; the second is a moderate but more longlasting stress. Our reactions to these two kinds of stresses tend to be different. In the first case we mobilize all of our energies to deal with the threatening situation but when the crisis passes we return to a more normal state. Short-term stress taxes our energies, but with time we are usually able to recover. In contrast, long term stress is usually more demanding. Instead of mobilizing our resources for a short burst of energy, we must resist for a long period. With little chance to rest and recover our strength, long term resistance can be very exhausting.

Reactions to stress are both physical and psychological; it should be remembered that the *whole* organism responds to stress. *The physical and psychological reactions occur together, not in isolation.*

Physical reactions to stress

Physical reactions to stress may occur in three stages. First, is the stage of "*alarm and mobilization.*" The heart beats faster, breathing becomes more rapid, digestive processes slow down, muscles become tense, and the individual becomes more alert.

These physical reactions enable the body to handle short-term stresses following which there is a relatively rapid return to a more normal physiological state. When the stress persists a stage of "*resistance*" begins in which the body prepares to cope with prolonged stress and attempts at the same time to maintain some kind of physiological balance. If the stress continues, strength eventually may be depleted, the individual is no longer able to resist and the stage of "*exhaustion*" and collapse occurs.

Recovery from the effects of such prolonged stress is often very slow (Torrance, 1965).

Psychological reactions to stress

The physiological stress reactions are accompanied by a number of psychological reactions. As little children, each of us learn how to cope with stress, but we don't all learn to cope in the same way (Murphy, 1962). Because of these different experiences in childhood, people differ in how they react to stress as adults, but it is possible to identify some common psychological reactions.

Task-directed reactions

In many stressful situations, we try to tackle the problem directly and handle it in a realistic way. To do so, we must define the problem, work out possible solutions, decide on the most suitable course of action and try it out. Sometimes more than one solution is tried before we find one which is effective.

The most common task-directed reactions are attack, withdrawal, and compromise. **Attack** involves an attempt to remove or surmount the stressful situation. The minister feels pressure because he does not have a sermon prepared but can attack the problem by locking himself in the study and working on the message. The prisoner of war who is under the stress of confinement might plan a method for escape.

When one moves to overcome a stress, the possibility of failure is always present. Attacking a problem, therefore, always involves taking a risk (Torrance, 1965). Of course, the risk is greater in some situations than in others. If the risk is small, attack may be a good way to handle a stress. If the risk is very great, attack might best be avoided. The prisoner of war, for example, may decide that he is likely to get caught and punished if he tries to escape. In such a case, attack may be too risky and too costly a solution to a problem.

Withdrawal can be either physical or psychological. The person who is losing an argument may leave the room (graciously if possible) or he may rely on such psychological techniques as changing the subject, admitting defeat, conveniently forgetting "what I was going to say," or suggesting that "we discuss this more later" in hopes that the subject will never come up again. By withdrawing from a stressful situation, the person is avoiding the difficulty.

Sometimes a total and permanent withdrawal is possible but even a temporary drawing apart can be helpful. By taking a short vacation, laying an issue aside for a while, or discussing it with a friend, often the individual can return to face the stress with new vigor and efficiency.

In writing this book, the author periodically finds that he cannot form words and phrases to express what he wants to say. At such times a short walk around the room, or a skimming over what has been written previously, provides a temporary withdrawal which is then followed (sometimes) by a new burst of ideas. Occasionally I leave the manuscript altogether for a while and go for coffee or for a time of browsing through a magazine. At such times there is, of course, the danger of being distracted and not returning to my work. If the task is to be completed withdrawal must be only temporary.

Compromise reduces the stress that comes from the changing of one's aspirations, expectations or activities. A student who is getting poorer grades than he expected may lower his aspirations and settle for C's. A husband and wife may make concessions to each other in order to bring better family relations. Likewise, disagreeing groups will sometimes arrive at a "bargain" in which each gives in a little to the other's demands.

"Compromise" is often thought of as something bad. Sometimes compromise does involve weakness and the lowering of one's standards, but at other times, compromise is *a wise and effective way* of handling stress.

Hope is another way of coping with the stresses of life. When he hopes, the individual takes "bits of reality" and ties them together by logic, reasoning and expectation (Korner, 1970; Frank, 1968). He has something to cling to, something that will keep him from despair and motivate him to press on in spite of the difficulties of the situation. Hope is an important characteristic for all men and especially for those who have hope because they are "in Christ" (Romans 15:13).

Then there is **prayer** and a reliance on the leading and intervention of God. For the Christian this is a crucial and a very practical way of tackling a difficult situation. The Christian believes that God hears and answers prayers, sometimes through divine intervention in stressful situations. At other times, the Holy Spirit guides men as they deal with their problems (John 16:13). Most psychology textbooks do not mention the influence of the supernatural, but this is a significant force in the life of the believer (Philippians 4:6, 7).

Defensive mechanisms

In dealing with the stresses of life we are sometimes unable or unwilling to tackle the problem directly. We may try to "hide" and we develop defensive ways of thinking which protect us from anxiety, soften failures, and preserve self-esteem. Psychologists call these ways of thinking **defensive mechanisms**; they are often unconscious reactions and rarely used deliberately.

Although psychologists have suggested as many as thirty defensive mechanisms, only a few are listed below. The church leader has seen many of these in himself and/or in his congregation.

Rationalization is the making of logically-sounding excuses in an attempt to justify something we have done or failed to do. We may be going 60 in a 40-kilometer-an-hour zone, but tell ourselves "it's okay because everyone else is doing it." The overweight lady may take a big dessert because "everyone should splurge once in a while." Sometimes Christians engage in sin and then rationalize their behavior by concluding "we must be 'one of the gang' if we are going to be a real witness for Christ."

Repression involves shutting out from our minds all those desires, impulses, thoughts, and ideas that are threatening. The church organist who plays a sour note during the offertory, or the young preacher who gives a poor sermon may put the memory of these unpleasant and embarrassing experiences out of their minds.

Regression occurs when an adult reacts to stress in a way which at an earlier time in life was successfully used to avoid unpleasant situations. When a new baby enters a home, older children sometimes return to baby talk or bed wetting in an attempt to get attention.

Projection involves blaming someone else for the motives and weaknesses that are really our own. A student who fails a test because of his lack of ability or preparation may push the blame on to the professor's "poor lectures" or the textbook's "lack of clarity." Intolerant church members usually deny their own lack of tolerance, but are quick to accuse members of other denominations of being rigid and intolerant.

Displacement often results as a response to frustration. Instead of directing our feelings toward the source of our frustrations, we channel feelings instead toward some less threatening person or object. The man who is bawled out by his boss may in turn "let off steam" by yelling at his secretary or wife.

Fantasy is a retreat from stressful reality and a move into some kind of dream world. Relaxing with a novel, watching a movie or television, or day-dreaming, are widely used fantasy activities.

Reaction formation is an attempt to hide or squelch one type of impulse by stressing the opposite. Sometimes people who are strongly attracted to sex magazines become militant crusaders against "obscene literature on our news-stands." Those who would really like to be dirty and messy sometimes are excessively neat and clean instead. In each of these situations, the person defends himself against his real feelings by stressing the opposite.

Identification involves taking on the characteristics of some person whom we admire. The young seminary student who is not doing very well in his first attempts at preaching may consciously or unconsciously imitate and take on the characteristics of some successful preacher whom he admires. Little children usually identify with their parents and sometimes parents identify with their successful children. In each case we reduce the stress of facing our own weaknesses by becoming like someone whom we see as being in a more desirable situation.

Malingering is the removal of stress by consciously or unconsciously feigning illness. When we are sick, we have a socially acceptable excuse for avoiding the stresses of life. If the stresses are especially intense, it may be handy to *appear* sick. This often has an added "fringe benefit." In addition to removal of unwanted stress, sickness can bring attention and sympathy.

Collapse. Sometimes, stress is so great that a person can neither deal with it, nor defend himself against it. In such situations, the individual "breaks down" and is no longer able to function efficiently.

ANXIETY AND STRESS

The twentieth century has been called "the age of anxiety." In the opinion of some psychologists, anxiety is "the official emotion" of our time and the emotion of "central significance" in all abnormal behavior (Levitt, 1967).

Anxiety is an emotional state resulting from stress and is characterized by apprehension, uneasiness, and fear. Sometimes anxiety arises when we are aware of a recognizable threat. At other times we feel anxious, but cannot find any reason for our feelings. Some people are anxious almost all the time; others are relatively free from anxiety, except in very stressful situations. Anxiety may be so intense that a person is immobilized, or it may be so mild that it is hardly noticed. It can be conscious or unconscious. It can interfere with our activities, as in stagefright, or it can spur us on to greater efforts, for example – anxiety about a test causes us to study harder. Apparently too little anxiety can be almost as harmful as too much.

The church leader is most likely to observe anxiety when he is visiting with the sick and their families. The prospect of surgery, the coming of death, and even the need to visit the dentist are stresses that can result in great anxiety. According to one psychologist who studied surgical patients,

> A major operation constitutes a stress situation which resembles many other types of catastrophes and disasters in that the "victim" faces a combination of three major forms of imminent danger – the possibility of suffering acute pain, of undergoing serious body damage, and of dying (Janis, 1958).

Presumably a similar pattern of anxiety occurs in the families of mental patients.

The church leader can bring comfort to anxious people such as these, reminding them that God is present and working even in the midst of stress and anxiety.

12

Stress in the Ministry

The minister and his family are not immune from the stress and anxiety that we discussed in the previous chapter. On the contrary, the ministry is characterized by a number of unique stresses. These include:

Social isolation The young Christian is applauded when he first declares his intention to enter the ministry and often respected as a leader when he later enters the pastorate. Like all people in public life, however, the minister has a *lonely job*. He lives in a fishbowl where he is carefully watched by the congregation. The pastor and his wife must listen to the problems of others - for this is an important part of their ministry - but there are few to whom they can confidentially express their own discouragements and uncertainties.

Excessive demands A pastor is expected to fulfill many roles: preacher, evangelist, youth leader, saint, scholar, father, counselor, parish promoter, community problem solver and (in many places) janitor, secretary, mimeograph operator - to name a few. His wife, often having little or no theological training, is expected to speak, make calls and generally fulfill the functions of assistant pastor. Even the pastor's children feel demands when they are expected to be well-behaved, strongly spiritual and present at all meetings of their age group. Too often, the many demands of his job rob the pastor of necessary time with God, interfere with family fellowship and bring feelings of anxiety, discouragement and inferiority.

Financial strain Even with fringe benefits, the pastor's family in many cases is forced to struggle along on a very tight budget. This can cause strain within the family circle and concern over the pressure of meeting financial obligations in a manner that will maintain one's good Christian witness. (Romans 12:17b, "Be careful to do what is right in the sight of everybody." This includes the prompt payment of debts or better yet the refusal to go into debt.)

Administrative pressures Church affairs must be conducted in an orderly manner (1 Corinthians 14:40) and a pastor is in overall charge of a big business. He is often responsible for efficient handling of a substantial budget, a detailed program and a church board that may not always be sympathetic or supportive. Since few seminaries or Bible schools provide training in good business methods, the pastor must struggle along as best he can, hoping that some members of the church will be able to give good business advice. All too frequently, these administrative demands take up so much time that the pastor is forced to reduce his study and prayer time. Increasing frustration develops as men who feel called to minister spend increasing amounts of time as administrators.

Professional competition Competition is a characteristic of life. Children compete for grades and athletic trophies. Merchants compete for sales. Politicians compete for votes. Military, professional and businessmen compete for advancement and increased assurances of security. It is hardly surprising then, that this attitude seeps into the ministry. Large building programs, large churches, large membership lists, large crowds, large budgets or large numbers of "decisions" sometimes become status symbols and objects of competition among pastors. Such competition detracts from the main function of the pastorate and is certain to produce frustration, jealousy and continued pressure in the lives of the competitors and their families.

Psychological tensions Discouragement is common among all Christians. It is especially easy for the pastor to get depressed when he considers the task that he is called to perform, the lethargy of so many Christians and the apparent lack of results.

Feelings of inadequacy, while common among pastors, present a special problem for the *pastors' wives* who rarely have any seminary or other training to prepare them for their roles.

Guilt sometimes arises because the pastor and his family are expected to be Christian leaders and examples. Like other Christians, however, they are tempted to sin, and sometimes they yield to these temptations. This easily leads to strong guilt feelings and a failure to accept God's wonderful forgiveness (1 John 1:9).

Anger is a psychological reaction that everyone experiences and a reaction that can often be constructive. In Mark 3:5

we read that Jesus was angry and He must have had the same feelings when He drove the money changers out of the temple. Often anger leads to harsh words, cynical comments, criticism and a lack of cooperation which only produce greater tension. Recently a pastor's wife wrote: "My husband is always too busy and too tired to spend time with me - much less the baby. I honestly feel that he doesn't care about the baby or me - but is in love with his books and the church and nothing else. I resent this! Why be married?"

Dealing with stress in the ministry

Like anyone else, the minister may react to stress. Like any other person, the minister or member of his family may experience a psychological breakdown or physical collapse if the stress is intense enough. Such breakdowns can be avoided, however, if the minister and the members of his congregation take certain precautions.

Have regular physical check-ups A close relationship exists between psychological and the physical functioning. For this reason, the pastor or the member of his family who is physically "run-down" or who suffers from some undetected physical defect is especially susceptible to pressures from his environment. Periodic physical examinations can lead to the recognition and probably elimination of physical disorders that could increase vulnerability to emotional breakdown.

In a very practical memo to pastors, one physician gave these "prescriptions for good health": get regular and vigorous exercise, do not become overweight, and avoid fatigue or stress.

Get organized With so many responsibilities and so many demands on his time, the pastor often finds that things begin to pile up. Instead of dealing with one matter at a time, he finds that it is easy to worry about everything at once. As a result, his concentration is divided and his efficiency is reduced. As he gets further behind, work gets done in a haphazard fashion and the pastor discovers that he is becoming more irritable, more discouraged and more susceptible to the pressures of his environment.

With a life of so many unexpected (and expected) interruptions, it is difficult for a pastor to organize his activities. Nevertheless, the following might be helpful suggestions. First *plan each day*. The pastor should decide what he would like to accomplish in a given time and set out to reach his goal. This will also involve advance planning as he decides on regular times for study, visitation, consultation, and administration. It may also involve educating the congregation to the fact that while he is always available for ministering to spiritual needs, the pastor would prefer to discuss church business or other matters during the times when he is available for consultation "in" his study. In planning time, however, the pastor should not be so rigid that he gets discouraged when he fails to finish all that he had hoped. This brings us to a second suggestion: *set realistic goals*. Moody is reported to have remarked one time that he "would rather put ten men to work than do the work of ten men." Jesus didn't try to carry on His work alone. He trained disciples and sent them out as co-laborers. The pastor who feels that he must shoulder all of the responsibility in the church might remember that while it may be the easiest way to get things done, it also encourages laziness and lethargy in his congregation and brings increased pressure into his own life. By setting realistic goals for himself and by encouraging others to help, the pastor obtains greater efficiency and emotional stability through better organization.

Take time to relax The minister should stop feeling guilty because he is "taking time away from the work" to which he feels called. A regular time set aside each week for rest and relaxation enables the pastor to carry on with renewed strength, enthusiasm and efficiency. If possible, at least some of this relaxation time should be spent with the family. This time may not be long, but at least it shows the pastor's wife that she is loved and appreciated, and it shows the children that "although daddy is busy, he still is our daddy."

Find a sympathetic friend At some time, every pastor needs a pastor. The ministry has many stresses and when one's emotions are ignored, they have a way of festering and producing additional psychological problems. By accepting and expressing their feelings and by sharing their burdens, the pastor and his wife can "let off steam" and learn to see themselves as others see them.

Utilize spiritual resources Ephesians 6 clearly shows that the Christian is in a serious battle with powerful Satanic forces. We must put on the whole armor of God and this involves being armed with the Word of God, supported by prayer, strengthened by the Holy Spirit and constantly alert. Like any busy professional it is easy for the pastor to become so engrossed in the cares of his occupation that he spends less and less time with his Lord. The devotional time can easily become a daily guilt-relieving ritual, rather than a vital time of strengthening through fervent prayer and close involvement with the Word of

God. Pastors need to remind themselves - as they remind their congregation - that the man who is too busy to study and spend time in prayer, *is too busy*!

The minister and his family should not shoulder all of the responsibility for dealing with pastoral pressures. The members of the congregation have a Christian responsibility to help the pastor as he faces the demands of the ministry to which he has been called. If church members would engage in the following, the pastor would be strengthened, his ministry would be more effective, the congregation would reap the benefits, and the church of Jesus Christ would take another surge forward.

Pray for the pastor The New Testament contains many examples of the power of prayer. This power is still available and the pastor who is backed by a praying congregation will have a more efficient and spiritually enriched ministry (see Ephesians 6:18).

Recognize the problems of the ministry Even very active church members often fail to recognize the burden that is faced by the average pastor. It is almost impossible for the pastor to talk openly about stress in the ministry - for he is sure to be misunderstood. Lay church leaders can alert the congregation to these problems, however, and this can hopefully lead church members to be less demanding and more considerate of the pastor and his family.

Remove some of the pressures In Acts we see murmuring in the church. Apparently the church leaders had become so busy that they could not meet all of their obligations. The problem was solved when church members took over some of the pastoral responsibilities.

By recognizing the pastor's strengths and helping where he is weak, the church members can do much to eliminate murmuring and help the pastor in his ministry. "Our pastor isn't very good at visiting and making calls," a lady once remarked to the author, "but his sermons are well prepared - and there are others of us in the church who can do the visiting." This is the spirit of understanding and cooperation which reduces pastoral tensions.

Provide an adequate salary The pastor should not be required to live on a salary which is below the average of his congregation. A good guideline in fixing the salary would be as follows. Invite all members of the church board to anonymously write their annual salary (before taxes) on a slip of paper. These figures could be added and averaged to arrive at a suitable salary for the pastor. There is a good chance that he would get a deserved raise!

Respect the pastor's personal life and study time Good sermons are not prepared in the midst of constant interruptions. The church members including the lay leaders should try to avoid disturbing the pastor when he is studying, should encourage the pastor to take at least one day off every week, and should try to respect the pastor's privacy.

Stress and the church

Groups and individuals within the church, including the pastor and his family, are all influenced by the stresses of modern living. The church leader who wants to understand behavior and work effectively with people must know something about the causes of stress and the ways in which people commonly react to the problems of life. Such knowledge enables the leader to (1) better understand and accept the actions of people who are experiencing stress; (2) identify individuals who are having difficulty in handling stress; (3) more effectively counsel with such people; (4) minister more helpfully to families at times of illness, death, and other crises; and (5) more easily handle the stresses which come into his own life and family.

Summary

Anxiety and psychological stress are almost universal in our modern society. When a situation hinders us, makes a task more difficult, or causes us to fail, we experience stress which is accompanied frequently by feelings of anxiety.

Most stress occurs when we are frustrated, in the midst of conflict or under some kind of pressure. The way people respond to these difficulties depends somewhat on the severity of the stress, but there are almost always both physical and psychological reactions.

Stress and anxiety is not confined to individuals such as church members. Groups sometimes come under stress and so do pastors and their families. When we know something about the causes of stress and typical stress reactions we are better able to minister to the people with whom we come in contact.

Notes

Chapter 1

1 H. J. Clinebell, Jr., *Basic Types of Pastoral Counseling.*
2 S. Freud, *The Problem of Lay-Analyses*, p. 11.
3 A. Benjamin, *The Helping Interview.*
4 J. S. Bonnell, *Psychology for Pastor and People*, p. 44.
5 C. M. Lowell, "Value Orientations - An Ethical Dilemma," *American Psychologist* 14 (1959): 687-93; Edith Weisskopf-Joelson, "Psychology and the Insights of Religion"; E.G. Williamson, "Value Orientation in Counseling" in *Humanistic Viewpoints in Psychology*, ed., F.T. Severin, pp. 359-77.
6 D. Johnson, *Marriage Counseling: Theory and Practice*, p. vii.
7 B. Shertzer and S.C. Stone, *Fundamentals of Counseling*, p. 157.
8 C.M. Narramore, *The Psychology of Counseling.*
9 D. H. Blocher, *Developmental Counseling.*
10 Benjamin.
11 E. H. Porter, Jr., *An Introduction to Therapeutic Counseling.*
12 D. F. Tweedie, *The Christian and the Couch.*
13 Narramore.
14 R. May, *The Art of Counseling*, p. 173.

Chapter 2

1 R. N. Robertson, L. T. Maholick and D. S. Shapiro, "The Parish Minister as Counselor: A Dilemma and Challenge," *Pastoral Psychology* 20 (June 1969): 24-30.
2 H. B. English and Ava C. English, *A Comprehensive Dictionary of Psychological and Psychoanalytical Terms*, p. 437.
3 H. J. Clinebell, Jr., *Basic Types of Pastoral Counseling*, p. 140.
4 Ibid.

5 J. Dollard and N. E. Miller, *Personality and Psychotherapy*; and R. Dayringer, "A Learning-Theory Approach to Pastoral Counseling," *Pastoral Psychology* 20 (Mar. 1969): 39-43.
6 S. Freud, *Civilization and Its Discontents*, P. 26.
7 W. B. Oglesby, Jr., *Referral in Pastoral Counseling.*
8 C. Reid, *Groups Alive - Church Alive.*
9 K. Miller, *A Second Touch*, p. 142.

Chapter 3

1 Joint Commission on Mental Illness and Health, *Action for Mental Health.*
2 M. P. Strommen, *Profiles of Church Youth*; R. B. Zuck and G. A. Getz, *Christian Youth: An In-Depth Study.*
3 H. J. Clinebell, Jr., *Basic Types of Pastoral Counseling*, p. 96.
4 L. M. Terman, *Psychological Factors in Marital Happiness.*
5 J. K. Morris, *Premarital Counseling: A Manual for Ministers*; and R. L. Dicks, *Premarital Guidance.*
6 K. R. Mitchell, "Reinterpreting the Purpose of Premarital Counseling," *Pastoral Psychology* 18 (Oct. 1967): 18-24.
7 J. R. Udry, *The Social Context of Marriage*; and J. C. Coleman, *Psychology and Effective Behavior.*
8 Ibid.
9 R. O. Blood, Jr., *Marriage*; J. Nederhood, *Too Early to Marry*; and J. C. Coleman, *Psychology and Effective Behavior.*
10 D. L. Womble, *Foundations for Marriage and Family Relations.*
11 P. H. Landis, *Making the Most of Marriage.*
12 Blood.
13 J. T. Landis, "Adjustments After Marriage; *Marriage and Family Living* 9(1947): 32-34.
14 Womble.

15 S. B. Babbage, *Sex and Sanity*: and B. L. Smith, "Till Death Us Do Part?" *Christianity Today* 14 (Jan. 16, 1970): 5-10).
16 Helpful books include: S. A. Lewin and J. Gilmore, *Sex Without Fear*; H. J. Miles, *Sexual Happiness in Marriage*; D. H. Small, *Design for Christian Marriage*; and R. B. Thieme, Jr., *The Biblical View of Sex, Love and Marriage.*
17 Clinebell, p. 98.
18 A. D. Bell, *The Family in Dialogue.*
19 W. L. Carrington, *The Healing of Marriage.*
20 Clinebell, p. 98.
21 W. C. Ellzey, "Education for the Newly Married," *Pastoral Psychology* 19 (May 1968: 21-26).
22 G. V. Ramsey, "Group Marriage Counseling for Normal Young Marrieds," *Pastoral Psychology* 13 (Mar. 1962): 30-34.
23 Blood.
24 R. L. Hudson, *Marital Counseling.*
25 Blood.
26 V. Satir, *Cojoint Family Therapy.*
27 Buker.

Chapter 4

1 M. Rosenburg, *Occupations and Values.*
2 R. B. Hackman, "Vocational Counseling with Adolescents" in *Understanding Adolescense*, ed., J. F. Adams, p. 384.
3 L. J. Bischof, *Adult Psychology.*
4 J. H. Dickerson, "The Pastor's Role with Job-Related Problems," *Pastoral Psychology* 12 (Sept. 1961): 29-30.
5 A. Richardson, *The Biblical Doctrine of Work.*
6 Wilma Donahue et al., "Retirement: The Emerging Social Pattern" in *Handbook of Social Gerontology*, C. Tibbits (ed.).
7 C. F. Kemp, *The Pastor and Vocational Counseling.*
8 Ibid.

Chapter 5

1 E. E. Bruder, "The Pastoral Ministry to the Mentally Ill," *Pastoral Psychology* 17 (1966): 23-27.
2 P. B. Maves (ed.), *The Church and Mental Health*, p. 189.
3 J. L. Christenson, *The Pastor's Counseling Handbook.*
4 H. J. Clinebell, Jr., *Mental Health Through Christian Community.*
5 J. E. Kilgore, *Pastoral Care of the Hospitalized Child.*
6 T. Howard, "What About Unwed Mothers?" *Christianity Today* 14 (Mar. 13, 1970): 11-12.
7 E. Kubler-Ross, *On Death and Dying.*
8 Ibid, p. 100.
9 Ibid, p. 123.
10 Ibid., and T. Shea, "New Seminar Helps Take the Sting Out of Death," *National Observer* (Jan. 5, 1970), p. 22.
11 C. C. Bachmann, *Ministering to the Grief Sufferer*, and E. N. Jackson, *For the Living.*
12 G. Gorer, *Death, Grief and Mourning*, p. 121.
13 W. M. Lamers, Jr., "Death, Grief, Mourning, the Funeral and the Child"; E. N. Jackson, *Telling a Child About Death*; and S. Wolff, *Children Under Stress.*
14 T. L. Duncan, *Understanding and Helping the Narcotic Addict.*
15 V. Kreyer, "Feelings of Handicapped Individuals," *Pastoral Psychology* 16 (June): 41-44.
16 S. L. Fink, "Crisis and Motivation: A Theoretical Model," *Archives of Physical Medicine and Rehabilitation* 48 (Nov. 1967).

Chapter 6

1 Reported in J.A. Knight, *Conscience and Guilt.* New York: Appleton-Century-Crofts, 1969, p. 119.

Chapter 7

1 See A. Adler, *Understanding Human Nature*. New York: Greenburg 1927.
2 P. Mullahy, *Oedipus Myth and Complex: A Review of Psychoanalytic Theory*. New York: Grove Press, 1948, p. 116.
3 K. Horney, *The Neurotic Personality of Our Time*. New York: Norton, 1937, p. 220.

Chapter 8

1 E. Kubler-Ross, *On Death and Dying*. New York: Macmillan, 1969.
2 I.L. Janes, et. al., *Personality: Dynamics, Development and Assessment*. New York: Harcourt, Brace & World, 1969, pp. 172-174.
3 J.R.W. Stott, "When Should a Christian Weep?" *Christianity Today*. Vol. 14, November 7, 1969, pp. 3-5.
4 Ibid.

Chapter 9

1 M.F. Hoffman, Homosexual: *Psychology Today* 3 (July 1969): 43-45, 70.
2 W. Bromberg, "Homosexuality" in *The Encyclopedia of Mental Health*, 3:747-63.
3 D.J. West, *Homosexuality*; and D.L. Farnsworth, "Sexual Aberrations," *Journal of Religion and Health* 7 (Oct. 1968): 350-57.
4 E. Rosen, and I. Gregory, *Abnormal Psychology*.
5 I.C. Coleman, and W. Broen, *Abnormal Psychology and Normal Life*.
6 Hoffman.
7 Anonymous "Letter from a Homosexual" *Christianity Today* 912 (March 1968) 547.
8 H.K. Jones, *Toward Christian Understanding of the Homosexual*.

Chapter 10

1 M. Jahoda, *Current Concepts of Positive Mental Health.* pp. 13-14, as quoted by Clinebell.
2 Erich Fromm, *The Sane Society.*
3 H.A. Bowman, "The Nature of Mental Health" in *Understanding Mental Health,* ed. R.I. Sutherland and B.K. Smith, p. 33.
4 G. Caplan "Prevention of Mental Disorders" in *The Encyclopedia of Mental Health* 5:1561.
5 Caplan.

Subject Index

The Rehabilitation of People With Spinal Cord Injury

Shanker Nesathurai, MD, MPH, FRCP(C)
Editor

Chief of Physical Medicine and Rehabilitation
Hamilton Health Sciences and St. Joseph's Hospital

Division Director of Physical Medicine and Rehabilitation
Professor of Medicine
Michael G. DeGroote School of Medicine
McMaster University

Lecturer in Physical Medicine and Rehabilitation
Harvard Medical School, Spaulding Rehabilitation Hospital

Printed in the United States of America

Publisher's Cataloging-in-Publication data
Nesathurai, Shanker, MD, MPH, FRCP(C).
The Rehabilitation of People With Spinal Cord Injury/Editor Shanker Nesathurai, MD, MPH, FRCP(C).

ISBN 978-0-9801171-0-3

First Printing, 2000

Contact Information:
AAP PUBLISHING
82 Fairlawn Street
Whitinsville, MA 01588 USA
phone: 508-234-4494
email: arbuckleacademicpub@gmail.com

Cover Art: Jason Laramie

Table of Contents

Notice: The indications and dosages of all drugs in this book have been recommended in the medical literature and conform to the practices of the general community. The medications described do not necessarily have specific approval by the Food and Drug Administration for use in the diseases and dosages for which they are recommended. The package insert for each drug should be consulted for use and dosage as approved by the FDA. Because standards for usage change, it is advisable to keep abreast of revised recommendations, particularly those concerning new drugs. Despite the best efforts of the contributors, editor and publisher, there is the possibility that there may be errors in the recommended dose and/or indication of any particular medication. In this context, clinicians are encouraged to independently ascertain the appropriateness of any recommendation related to the dose and indication of a pharmacological treatment.

This book is dedicated to my wife Nancy and our precious children, Anne, Allan and Claire.

Introduction

A rehabilitation physician faces no greater challenge than coordinating the care of a patient with a spinal cord injury (SCI). To achieve optimal outcomes, the practitioner must understand both the biological and sociomedical issues. SCI clinicians must become adept at navigating through the arcane and complex public and private programs that may help their patients. On occasion, the programs designed to help persons with SCI have perverse incentives, which may impair social and vocational reintegration. Rehabilitation clinicians should also be cognizant of the architectural and attitudinal barriers that affect community reintegration. Spinal cord injury may not only profoundly impair the affected individual's functional independence; it also places a significant emotional and financial burden on both families and society. Despite these profound challenges, most people with SCI live satisfying and productive lives, with the support of friends and family.

For optimal outcomes, it is necessary to have a dedicated and knowledgeable team of physicians, nurses and therapists. This book is intended to provide an overview of the clinical issues for resident physicians. However, other members of the health-care team may find the monograph of interest. It provides guidelines for evaluation and management, but is by no means a comprehensive textbook. Often, the management strategies outlined reflect the practices and preferences of the contributors. As always, treatment decisions must be individualized.

Many of the topics discussed in this book have not been examined in a rigorous scientific manner. In some cases, the concepts presented are conceptualizations that assist in understanding a complex topic. For example, in this monograph, there are references to sacral and pontine micturition. It has not been definitively demonstrated, however, that these centers exist. In this context, the contributors hope that the readers will be inspired to organize and participate in studies that will contribute to scientific understanding.

The response to and comments about this monograph have been overwhelming. As such, this third edition contains a number of updates and revisions, including an additional chapter related to community reintegration in Canada. For more information on spinal cord injury, the contributors and editor recommend reviewing the suggested readings, which are in Appendix 1.

Although care has been taken with regard to the indications, contraindications and doses of interventions, the final responsibility rests with the prescribing practitioner. The therapeutic and adverse effects of certain medications may be greater in persons with SCI. As such, the maximum recommended doses of some drugs in this monograph may be lower than what is generally accepted in other populations. The readers are advised to critically review any treatment recommendations and, if necessary, refer to appropriate reference literature (e.g., Physicians' Desk Reference, American Hospital Formulary Service Drug Information Manual).

In the text, impairment of all four limbs has been categorized as *tetraplegia*, not quadriplegia. As well, skin breakdown has been labeled as *pressure ulcers* as opposed to the commonly used term decubitus ulcers. At present, tetraplegia and pressure ulcers are the preferred nomenclature.

Two of the chapters in the monograph were originally written by the late Dr. Allan Meyers, a thoughtful scholar who mentored a plethora of young faculty members. His chapters have been updated by Dr. Andrew Graham and Dr. Paul Stacey.

Again, the contributors welcome the comments and criticisms of the readers. These suggestions can be incorporated into future editions.

Shanker Nesathurai, MD, MPH, FRCP(C)
Hamilton, Ontario, Canada

Acknowledgments

The conceptualization, production and distribution of the first and second editions of this book were financially supported, in part, by a grant from the National Institute on Disability and Rehabilitation Research (NIDRR) to the New England Regional Spinal Cord Center at Boston Medical Center. Many of the contributors to this monograph continue academic and professional affiliations with current and former National Model Systems Centers. The chapter authors and editor are exceedingly grateful for the encouragement of Toby Lawrence and Dr. Joel Mykelbust, both of whom served as project officers at NIDRR.

This edition was financially supported by the Bay Area Health Trust, which is located in Hamilton, Canada. The Bay Area Health Trust's mission is to provide financial support to advance the clinical and research initiatives of Hamilton Health Sciences Group of Hospitals, as well as McMaster University's Faculty of Health Sciences. The contributors and editor are grateful for the assistance and support of Ms. Elizabeth Manganelli, president of the Bay Area Health Trust.

The contributors are grateful for the thoughtful and insightful criticisms of our colleagues. The following clinicians reviewed the manuscript and provided suggestions and recommendations related to this and/or previous editions of this monograph: Drs. Chunbo Cai, David Chen, Mel Glenn, Robert Krane (deceased), Radha Vijayakumar, Emilia Semenov, Karen Smith, Shahzad Tanwir and Buck Woo, and Ms. Kim Eberhart. Drs. Fred Maynard and David Apple and Ms. Leslie Hudson provided considerate advice with regard to ASIA scoring. Law professor Ilene Klein kindly reviewed the section on Social Security, Medicare and Medicaid benefits. Many of their suggestions were incorporated in the final text. The authors are also grateful to Scott Edwards, Patricia Regan, Wendy Locke and Marjorie Scott for their editorial assistance and Lisa Greenleaf for her art direction, design, and typesetting. The original artwork was prepared by Edward Skawinski, Richard Francey, and Jason Laramie.

Although the contributors are gratified by the support their respective institutions have provided, the opinions and comments expressed in this monograph are those of the authors. The opinions articulated are not endorsed by any organization, agency or reviewer.

Contributors

Dain Allred, MD
Private Practice
Colorado Springs, Colorado

Amy Bjornson, MPT, ATP
Private Practice
Sydney, Australia

Susan Biener Bergman, MD
Associate Clinical Professor of Rehabilitation Medicine
Boston University School of Medicine

Nancy DeSantis, DO
Assistant Professor of Medicine
Oakland University William Beaumont School of Medicine

Ada Dominguez, MD, FRCP(C)
Assistant Clinical Professor of Physical Medicine and Rehabilitation
McMaster University

Stanley Ducharme, PhD
Clinical Professor of Urology
Boston University School of Medicine

Florin Feloiu, MSc (PT), MSc (Kinesiology), MD
Senior Resident in Physical Medicine and Rehabilitation
McMaster University

Douglas Garland, MD
Clinical Professor of Orthopedic Surgery
University of Southern California

Mary Glover, MS, RNC
Director
Boston's Community Medical Group

Andrew Graham, PhD
Research Coordinator
McMaster University

Andrew Gwardjan, MD, FRCP(C)
Assistant Clinical Professor of Medicine
McMaster University

Anantha Kamath, MD
Private Practice
Atlanta, Georgia

Mark Kaplan, MD
Associate Clinical Professor of Orthopedics and Rehabilitation Medicine
University of Massachusetts Medical School

Dinesh Khumbare, MD, FRCP(C)
Associate Clinical Professor of Physical Medicine and Rehabilitation
McMaster University

Jim McCormack
President
Seaside Associates

Allan R. Meyers, PhD (deceased)
Research Professor of Rehabilitation Medicine
Boston University School of Medicine
Professor of Health Services
Boston University School of Public Health

Shanker Nesathurai, MD, MPH, FRCP(C)
Professor of Medicine
McMaster University
Lecturer in Physical Medicine and Rehabilitation
Harvard Medical School

Steven Nussbaum, MD
Assistant Professor of Rehabilitation Medicine
Northwestern University
Medical School

Adriano Persi, BSc. Pharm, DC
Assistant Adjunct Clinical Professor of Physical Medicine and Rehabilitation
McMaster University

J. Scott Richards, PhD
Professor of Physical Medicine and Rehabilitation
University of Alabama at Birmingham
School of Medicine

Elizabeth Roaf, MD
Assistant Professor of Orthopedics and Rehabilitation Medicine
University of Massachusetts Medical Center

John Sledge, MD
Private Practice
Lafayette, Louisiana

Paul Stacey, MD
Senior Resident in Physical Medicine and Rehabilitation
McMaster University

Jane Wierbicky, RN, BSN
Marblehead, Massachusetts

Chapter 1

The Epidemiology of Spinal Cord Injury

*Allan R. Meyers**
Andrew Graham
Paul Stacey

Introduction

For all of the concerns about the enduring medical, social, psychological and financial consequences of spinal cord injury (SCI), little is known about the epidemiology. Moreover, much of the epidemiologic knowledge is derived from local, regional or single-state studies that are as much as 40 years old. In some notable cases, the studies are inconsistent with one another. The available studies rely upon a variety of different research methods, including hospital discharge summaries, state registries, and specialized databases such as those maintained by the Department of Veterans Affairs (VA) and the National Model Spinal Cord Injury System (NMS). Even the most comprehensive databases may not be representative of all people with SCI. For example, the NMS database is estimated to include as many as 13 percent of all prevalent SCI. This is the most robust database related to SCI and is a data set for many systematic studies of SCI epidemiology. In addition, the NMS database is the source for most of the data in this chapter; however, it is challenged by high levels of missing data on some of the most epidemiologically vital aspects of SCI. Moreover, the NMS database is limited to adults who survive SCI, consent to inclusion in the database, and receive treatment at an NMS center; most participating institutions are academic medical centers which may manage a more severely injured SCI population. Most of the material in this chapter relates to the US experience with spinal cord injury; however, there is some additional information related to the Canadian experience, as well.

There have been significant improvements in the collection and analysis of SCI data. Public and private agencies, such as the Centers for Disease Control and Prevention (CDC), the US Department of Education's National Institute on Disability and Rehabilitation Research (NIDRR), and the Paralyzed Veterans of America (PVA), have provided funding for some extremely interesting and useful research. For example, the CDC has sponsored the development and implementation of a number of state SCI registries. The VA has established a national registry of spinal cord dysfunction that includes traumatic SCI. At the same time, none of our national data programs systematically report or record SCI, nor are they likely to do so in the foreseeable future. State registries have had limited success recording and tracking those injured. Despite the growing corpus of research and number of investigators, there continue to be basic questions about the epidemiology of SCI which have not been definitively answered.

*Deceased

Incidence, Prevalence, and Survival

With these caveats noted, the annual incidence rate appears to be about 30 to 40 new injuries per million people per year, although some local and regional studies suggest rates as high as 60 per million people per year. These figures refer only to survivors. Although there has been a trend toward improved survival and increased longevity for people with traumatic SCI, the data suggests that there are about 10 to 20 fatal injuries per million people per year; that is, injuries resulting either in immediate death or death before hospital admission. There is considerable evidence for changes in cause-specific incidence rates, but little evidence that overall incidence rates have changed in the past 30 years.

In 2009, the number of people in the United States who were living with a spinal cord injury was estimated to be approximately 270,000, with a range of 236,000 to 327,000. There is considerable evidence that acute and long-term survival has increased due to improved health-care services and assistive technologies. Persons with SCI are living many decades after their initial injuries and now suffer from many of the same diseases that afflict individuals without SCI (i.e., cardiovascular disease, stroke, diabetes, cancer, etc.). Further advances in treatment may also decrease mortality in the SCI population and further increase the prevalence rate.

Characteristics of Injuries

The NMS database contains the largest and most consistent data on the neurological and anatomical characteristics of SCI in the US. The database includes information related to the time of initial (emergency) admission, initiation of acute rehabilitation programs, as well as post-discharge environment. The National Spinal Cord Injury Database includes cases from the US since 1973 and, as of October 2009, contains information on 28,450 persons. Their data suggest that, at discharge, the most prevalent neurological levels are C5 (16 percent), C4 (13 percent), C6 (13 percent), T12 (8 percent), C7 (6 percent), and L1 (5 percent). The most recent data suggests that approximately 55 percent of patients in the database are classified as having tetraplegia and 45 percent are classified as having paraplegia.

Some state and local SCI registries and other data sources show somewhat different prevalence rates, generally with higher rates of lower-level lesions. This variation may be secondary to local cultural or behavioral patterns (e.g., higher frequencies of gunshot wounds in southern and southwestern states). An alternate explanation may be that people with lower-level lesions are less likely to receive treatment in academic centers and, therefore, are less likely to be enrolled in the NMS database.

There has been an overall decrease in the percentage of patients reported to the database as clinically complete versus incomplete. From 1981 to 1992, 52 percent of reported injuries were complete and 48 percent were incomplete. Since 2005, approximately 40 percent were reported as complete at discharge and approximately 60 percent were incomplete.

Comorbid Injuries

For obvious reasons, SCI are catastrophic outcomes in their own right. Nevertheless, many people with SCI (55 percent of those in the NMS database) experience comorbid injuries whose consequences and secondary conditions may be as clinically,

psychologically and socially significant as SCI. Among these, the most prominent recorded in the NMS database are fractures (sites unspecified; 29 percent of all SCI), head injury (12 percent; although an additional 28 percent report "loss of consciousness"), and pneumothorax or hemothorax (18 percent).

Demographics: Age, Gender, Marital Status, Ethnicity, Education, Employment, and Race

Though there may be important age-related reporting biases affecting both children and older adults, those at highest risk of SCI appear to be around 40 years of age. There has been an increase in the average age of injured persons, from 28.7 years from 1973 to 1979 to 40.2 years since 2005. Children (15 years or younger) account for only 4.5 percent of cases; older adults (those 75 years of age and older), only about 1 percent. As noted, these data should be interpreted with caution. At one age extreme, the NMS does not systematically enroll children (who cannot give independent informed consent) and, therefore, may be under-represented. At the opposite extreme, the under-representation of older adults may reflect differences in incidence, survival or both. It is also possible that many elderly patients with SCI are treated at non-NMS centers. As the population ages, the numbers of older adults with SCI should increase, even if there is no change in survival.

The association with gender is clear; more than 80 percent of those enrolled in the NMS database are males. Other databases confirm that males are more likely to suffer from SCI . There also is a close association between risk of SCI and a number of indicators of social class, all of which have profound implications for rehabilitation. For example, individuals with SCI have fewer years of education than their uninjured counterparts. They also are more likely than their uninjured counterparts to have been unemployed and to have been single (i.e., never married, separated or divorced).

There has been a significant change in the race/ethnicity of injured persons in the database. Since 2005, 66.2 percent were Caucasian, 14.2 percent were African American, and 2.0 percent were Asian. Prior to 1980, 20 percent of injuries were to African Americans.

Cause of Injury

As of 2005, vehicular crashes still account for the majority of SCI, representing 41.3 percent. There has been a decrease in the proportion of injuries caused by sports, from 13 percent to 7.9 percent, and violence, from 17 percent to 15 percent since 2005.

The number of SCI reported with other/unknown causes has remained relatively unchanged, from 8 percent prior to 1980 to 8.5 percent since 2005.

There are close relationships among injury etiology, age, gender and, perhaps, ethnicity. Although it is not possible in such a brief review to develop these concepts in adequate detail, younger males, in general, are more likely to experience sports-related injuries, and lower-income minority males are more likely to experience injuries related to violence.

Time of Injury: Season, Day and Hour

Consistent with the premise that injuries are not accidents, SCI appear to be clustered by season, day of the week, and time of day. Though seasonal trends tend to be less noteworthy in regions of the country characterized by less temperature fluctuation, there

is a clear summer peak, with the highest incidence in July. There also is a strong tendency for SCI to occur at night and on weekends: 20 percent of all SCI in the NMS database occur on Saturday nights. These trends are most notable for injuries that are associated with motor vehicle collisions and sports.

Alcohol, Drugs and SCI

Though there is substantial evidence of the roles of alcohol use and the use of other drugs (both legal and illegal) in trauma-related mortality and morbidity, there is little specific information about their effects on the incidence of SCI. Moreover, drug and substance screening are not completed routinely and consistently in emergency departments. In addition, the biochemical markers of many cognitively clouding compounds (i.e., alcohol) are highly transitory. As such, causal connections between SCI and substance consumption are very difficult to establish.

Other Risk-Factors: Psychology, Speed and Protective Equipment

As in the cases of alcohol and drug use, it is reasonable to infer that such factors as speed (in recreational, occupational and motor vehicle settings) and the use of safety equipment (i.e., seat belts and helmets) may affect the epidemiology of SCI. In addition, psychological traits, such as "locus-of-control" and "risk-taking," may affect the incidence of spinal cord injuries. However, there is little scientific evidence documenting such associations. It has been clearly demonstrated that mandatory seat belt and helmet statutes, in addition to vigorous enforcement of speeding and drunk driving laws, have reduced overall mortality. Efficacy of these interventions in reducing SCI, however, has not been studied. Increased survival of acute SCI, even when associated with a decreased incidence of MVC, may result in increased overall prevalence of SCI.

Epidemiology of Spinal Cord Injury in Canada

There are few rigorous studies reporting the incidence and prevalence of SCI in Canada. Extrapolating from data published by Noonan, et al., in 2012, the incidence of SCI is estimated at 109 cases per million. The prevalence is estimated to be approximately 2,600 cases per million. These figures aggregate both traumatic and non-traumatic cases. The number of traumatic and non-traumatic cases is approximately equal. Based on data published by Picket, et al., the most common causes of traumatic SCI in Canada are motor vehicle collisions and falls, which account for 35 percent and 32 percent, respectively. Less common causes of traumatic SCI include injuries associated with the use of bicycles, motorcycles and all-terrain vehicles; collectively, these injuries account for approximately 12 percent of SCI. Sports-related injuries and interpersonal violence account for an estimated 9 percent and 5 percent of SCI, respectively. A national Registry of Spinal Cord Injury is now being developed and implemented by hospitals across Canada. This registry will hopefully provide a more accurate assessment related to the epidemiology of SCI in Canada.

Conclusion

The three classic components of the epidemiologic triad are agent, vector and host. The characteristics of the hosts (the people who survive SCI) are most understood. Much less is known about the factors of agency and vector: matters related to protective (or

destructive) equipment; social contexts of drinking, driving, work and leisure; and facility design. Knowledge about the demographic characteristics (i.e., age, gender, race) of the hosts is most complete. However, most of these factors are not amenable to intervention. The least is known about host characteristics (i.e., risk-taking behavior, excessive speed, use of protective equipment) that may be influenced by public policy initiatives. If our goal is an epidemiology that serves the purposes of prevention, as opposed to description or prediction, then new questions must be asked, and better data must be collected. Toward that goal, informed and sensitive clinicians have a critical role.

Chapter 2

Pathophysiology of Spinal Cord Injury

Jane Wierbicky
Anantha Kamath

Anatomy

The spinal cord is a complex organized mass of nerve tissues that extends distally from the level of the occiput to approximately the L2 vertebra. It is located within the vertebral canal and surrounded by the meninges.

A cross-sectional view of cord tissue reveals the butterfly-shaped gray matter surrounded by white matter. The gray matter is symmetrical and comprised of anterior, lateral and posterior horns. The gray matter is principally composed of neuronal cell bodies, but also includes dendrites, axons and glial cells (e.g., oligodendrocytes, astrocytes, etc.). The anterior horn is comprised of the cell bodies of the motor neurons. The cell bodies of the preganglionic neurons of the sympathetic nervous system are located in the lateral horn. The cell bodies of sensory fibers, which are located in the dorsal root ganglion, project into the posterior horn.

The white matter is composed of longitudinal nerve fiber tracts amid a network of neuroglia. These fibers are either myelinated or nonmyelinated and allow communication between the spinal cord and the brain. The anterior, lateral and posterior columns of the white matter each contain ascending and descending tracts.

Each of the 31 pairs of spinal nerves contain thousands of nerve fibers that branch out from the spinal cord. Each spinal nerve is composed of a dorsal and a ventral root that unite in the vicinity of the intervertebral foramen. The dorsal root conveys sensory input to the cord, and the ventral root conveys motor impulses to the skeletal muscles. The ventral root also contains efferent visceral fibers, which conduct impulses to the involuntary smooth muscles and glands of the autonomic nervous system.

Mechanism of Injury

Traumatic, nonpenetrating injury to the spinal cord generally occurs by one, or a combination, of the following mechanisms: flexion, extension, rotation or vertical compression. These actions create an external force causing the displacement of the vertebral column and consequent compression of the cord parenchyma. This traumatic event may result in vertebral fracture and/or dislocation, injury to vascular components, or ligamentous disruption or rupture. The damage to the spinal cord parenchyma is classified as concussion, contusion or laceration (including transection).

A concussion is characterized by transient neurological symptoms with rapid resolution of deficits. No notable gross anatomic lesions are identifiable, and true cord concussion is rarely seen.

Cord contusion is frequently encountered in traumatic SCI. Classically, it is the result of the compression of the spinal cord. Although the gross structural continuity of the cord remains intact, the cord is bruised in appearance. This is a result of petechial hemorrhage into surrounding tissues.

Cord lacerations are the result of severe displacements of the vertebral column. The bony fragments of vertebral fractures may retropulse into the spinal canal and thereby cause grossly visible laceration or disruption of the cord tissues. Traumatic intervertebral disc herniations could impinge upon the spinal cord and associated vasculature. Membranes may be torn and, in some instances, the cord may be completely transected. Due to the ensuing damage to the motor, sensory and autonomic pathways, there may be partial or complete loss of function below the level of the lesion.

Missile Injuries to the Spinal Cord

The extent of tissue injury sustained from a missile wound is directly related to the mass and velocity of the projectile. As a bullet passes through tissue, a wound track is formed. The structures that are immediately adjacent to this track (i.e., bone and ligaments) are displaced with such speed and force that they themselves act as secondary missiles. Bullets may fragment and ricochet, which can increase the amount of neurological injury. Retained missile fragments may cause a foreign body reaction in the spinal cord. In addition, there is a high incidence of infection. Antibiotics and tetanus toxoid should be considered.

Progression of Lesion Development in Moderate and Severe SCI

A secondary chain of cellular events is set into motion immediately following the initial insult to the spinal cord. The pathophysiology of the injury can be divided into three stages: acute, intermediate and late.

Acute Stage

Inflammatory reactions (i.e., edema, hyperemia, hemorrhage) of the spinal cord may develop immediately post-injury. The cell membranes are highly permeable in the acute stage, and edema may be present up to 15 days post-injury. The endothelial cells of the intact capillaries become edematous, thereby limiting perfusion and resulting in ischemia. There may be further risk of ischemic damage in persons experiencing hypovolemic shock or those requiring cardiopulmonary resuscitation. Damage to the spinal vasculature and thrombosis may also result in further ischemia.

Monocytes are mobilized from the damaged vessels and are eventually converted to macrophages. The macrophages will begin their phagocytic role in the gray matter of the cord and remove necrotic debris from the area of injury. This process of phagocytosis will continue until the debris is removed and a central cavity develops. Nerve compromise is manifested by traumatic demyelination and fragmentation changes of the axonal cylinders. Vacuoles may develop in the white matter secondary to the breakdown of the myelin sheaths surrounding the axons. After several days, glial cells proliferate, forming astrocytic fibers between the necrotic cavity and the intact tissue. These cavities, which represent sites of complete parenchymal hemorrhagic necrosis, may be singular or multilocular.

Intermediate Stage

After several weeks, the cavity is fully developed and gliosis is complete. The edema has resolved and the cord appears atrophied. The meninges have become fibrotic, and the subarachnoid space at the level of the injury is sometimes obliterated. Anterior and posterior nerve root regeneration becomes apparent.

Late Stage

Several months post-injury, the cyst wall is thick. Collagenous fibrosis is present in varying degrees and is generally proportional to the degree of initial hemorrhage. Arachnoiditis may develop due to scarring of the membranes. In many cases, there is a degree of preserved white matter at the periphery of the lesion. Nerve root regeneration is present in most cases within one year post-injury.

Numerous complications may be encountered several years post-injury. Post-traumatic syringomyelia develops in 5 percent of the SCI population. Although the exact mechanism is unclear, chronic mechanical stress to the spinal cord (i.e., kyphosis, canal stenosis) may contribute to the development of a syrinx (see chapter 16). This post-traumatic cyst may progressively ascend or descend over many segments of the spinal cord. There may be a decrease in neurological function noted, and surgery to drain the cyst may be warranted. Osteoarthritis may also lead to further neurological decline. Osteophytes and herniated disks may impinge upon the spinal cord vasculature, impairing blood flow and resulting in ischemic changes. Traumatic neuromas arising from the spinal nerve roots are also occasionally encountered.

Non-Traumatic SCI

Non-traumatic SCI includes damage to the spinal cord in the absence of trauma. It can be caused by infection, cancer or ischemia, as well as by degenerative diseases of the spinal column. It has been estimated that non-traumatic SCI may affect two to three times more people than traumatic SCI.

Conclusion

The pathophysiology of traumatic spinal cord injury is complex and cannot be fully summarized in this brief review. In addition, many biological aspects of SCI warrant further investigation. An understanding of the concepts, however, provides a useful foundation for clinical practice.

Chapter 3

Surgical Management of Spine Fractures

John Sledge
Dain Allred

In the United States, spinal cord injuries are usually treated in tertiary care centers. Proper acute management requires the skills of a trauma team that is composed of nurses, emergency room physicians, general surgeons, orthopedic surgeons, neurological surgeons, and anesthesiologists. Rehabilitation clinicians, although not intimately involved with the emergent management, must have a basic understanding of the acute medical and surgical issues.

Figure 3.1 Human Spine

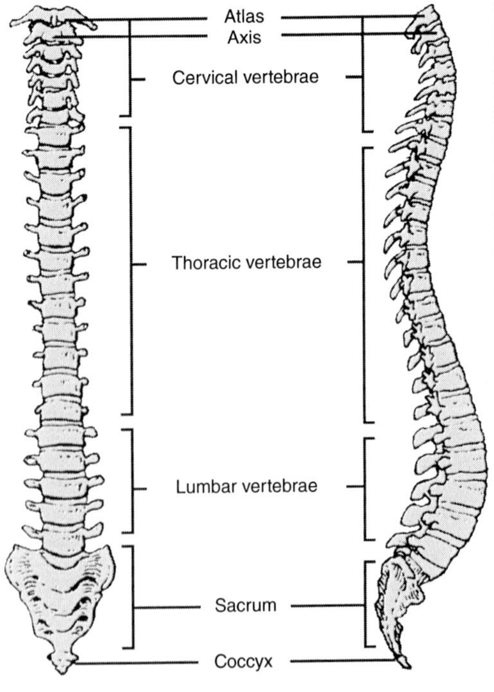

Anatomy

The spine has seven cervical vertebrae, 12 thoracic vertebrae, five lumbar vertebrae, and five sacral vertebrae (Figures 3.1, 3.2 and 3.3). The sacral vertebrae are fused. The spine allows for motion and provides strong protection for the spinal cord. The terminal portion of the spinal cord is the conus medullaris, which becomes the cauda equina ("horse's tail") at approximately the L2 vertebral level.

Clinical Evaluation

When a patient is involved in a significant trauma, an SCI should be suspected. A thorough clinical examination must be completed and lateral cervical spine X-ray must be ordered. Approximately 5 percent of patients with a spine injury will have a noncontiguous second lesion. If SCI cannot be excluded with

Figure 3.2 **C1 and C2 Vertebrae**

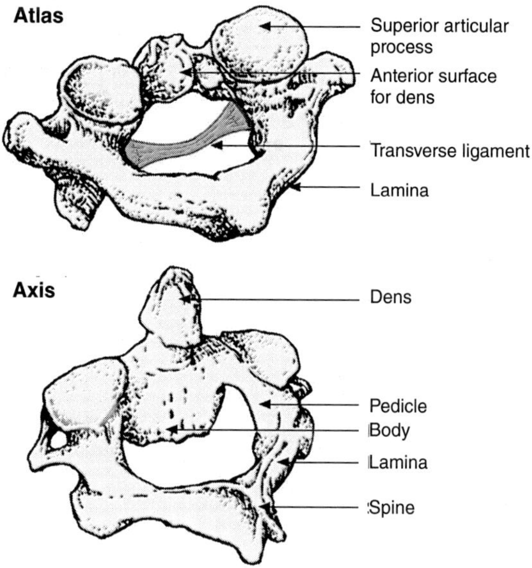

standard films, then further investigations, including flexion-extension views, CT scans or MRI studies should be completed. Unrecognized SCI can result in devastating clinical and medicolegal consequences.

The spine surgeon is concerned with the following issues. First, has the patient been appropriately resuscitated and stabilized (i.e., airway, breathing, circulation)? Second, is there a spinal injury and, if so, what type of injury is present? Third, does the patient have any neurological deficit secondary to spinal cord compromise (i.e., contusion, transection)? Fourth, on the basis of clinical examination, injury pattern and radiological studies, is the injury stable or unstable? Finally, is the treatment operative or non-operative (i.e., collar, SOMI brace, halo)? If the injury is unstable or there is neurological compromise, surgical intervention should be considered. The nature of the injury will determine whether operative intervention will be from an anterior or posterior approach, or both. The type of injury will also dictate if operative treatment involves decompression, instrumentation and/or fusion. The timing of surgery in an unstable injury with neurological deficits is somewhat controversial. Some would argue that surgery should be delayed until spinal cord edema has diminished; others believe delay in definitive treatment is unnecessary. Although treatment must be individualized, the following are some general guidelines for surgical management.

Figure 3.3 **Cervical, Thoracic & Lumbar Vertebrae**

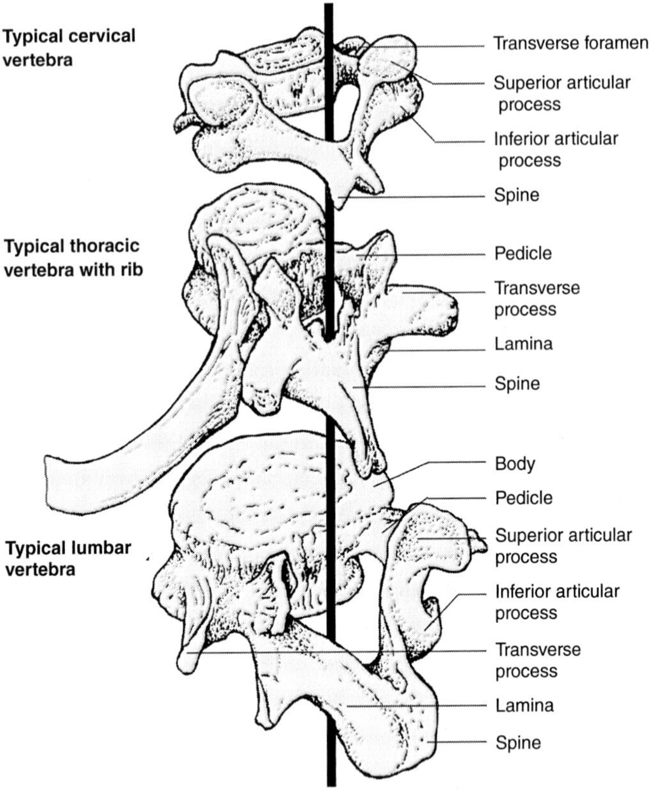

Pharmacological and Cellular Therapies

The National Acute Spinal Cord Injury 2 (NASCIS 2) study randomized non-penetrating acute SCI patients to placebo, high-dose methylprednisolone or naloxone. Patients with exclusively cauda equina lesions (i.e., L3 burst fracture) and penetrating wounds (i.e., gunshot injuries or stabbings) were excluded. Patients were enrolled within 12 hours of injury. Those assigned to the steroid arm received a bolus of 30 mg/kg, with a continuous infusion of 5.4 mg/kg/hr for 23 hours. Overall, there was no difference among the three treatment arms. There was, however, a reported benefit among those patients treated within eight hours of injury.

NASCIS 3 randomized SCI patients to 24 hours of methylprednisolone, 48 hours of methylprednisolone, or tirilazad mesylate. Again, there was no significant difference

among the three treatment arms when all patients were considered. However, 48 hours of methylprednisolone was reported to benefit those patients treated within three to eight hours of injury.

The statistical analysis and clinical significance of the putative gains attributed to methylprednisolone in both of these studies are not universally accepted. However, treatment with methylprednisolone is commonly accepted practice in Canada and the United States.

A clinical study evaluating the benefit of thyrotropin-releasing hormone (TRH) in acute spinal cord injury was completed in the early 1990s. The results suggested that there may be a positive role for TRH; however, only 20 patients were enrolled in the study and a number of patients were lost to follow up. At present, TRH cannot be recommended to treat acute SCI. GM-1 ganglioside (Sygen) has also been evaluated in clinical trials. Overall, this treatment has not been demonstrated as efficacious in the treatment of acute SCI. There have been reports in the scientific literature and lay media related to cellular therapies, including embryonic and fetal stem cells. Currently, the evidence is not convincing that these treatments are effective in treating acute SCI.

Spine Stability

In general, the stability of fractures of the occipital condyle, atlas (C1) and axis (C2) are determined by fracture pattern. Spinal stability of fractures of the lower cervical spine (C3 to C7) can be assessed by the criterion described by White and Punjabi. This system requires assessment of translation and angulation in cervical flexion and extension films. In general, relative sagittal plane translation of 3.5 mm is associated with instability. Likewise, relative sagittal plane angulation of greater than 11 degrees is associated with instability.

The stability of thoracic and lumbar injuries is evaluated by utilizing the three-column model described by Denis (Figure 3.4). The anterior column consists of the anterior longitudinal ligament, anterior vertebral body, and anterior annulus fibrosis. The middle column consists of the posterior vertebral body, posterior annulus fibrosis, posterior longitudinal ligament and spinal cord. The posterior column includes the spinous process, laminae, facets, pedicles and posterior ligamentous structures (i.e., ligamentum flavum, intraspinous ligaments, supraspinous ligaments). Fractures are deemed stable if there is compromise to only one column. The spine is considered unstable when two or more columns are compromised.

Cervical Spine Injuries

Occipital Condyle Injuries

Occipital condyle injuries are rare and can be classified into three different groups. Type 1 injuries are impaction injuries secondary to axial loading. Type 2 injuries are associated with basal skull fractures. Type 1 and Type 2 fractures are stable and can be treated with a cervical orthosis (i.e., Philadelphia collar, SOMI brace). Type 3 injuries are secondary to violent lateral or rotational forces and are associated with alar ligament avulsion. If there is instability, operative treatment is required.

Figure 3.4 **Three-Column Model of Spine Stability**

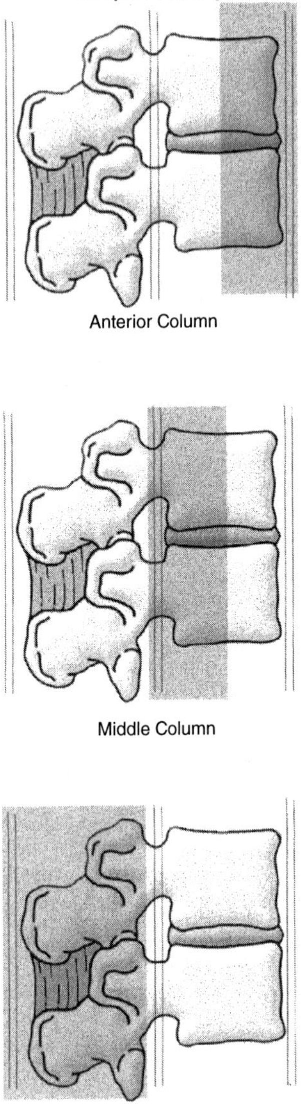

Figure 3.5 **C1 (Atlas) Fractures**

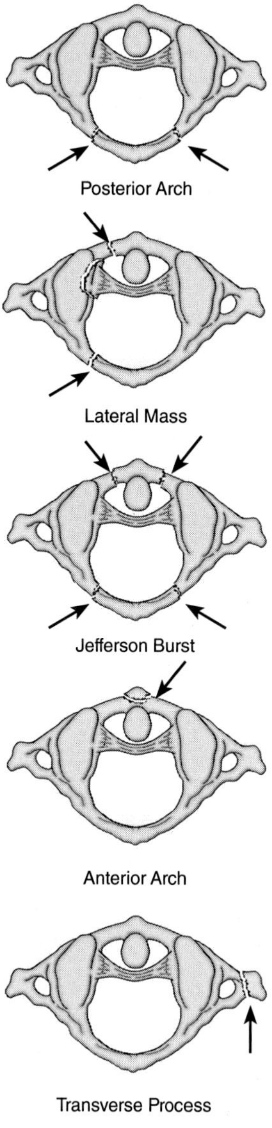

Posterior Arch Fracture

- Mechanism: combined extension and lateral loading
- Treatment: stable injury; initial treatment with cervical collar or halo

Lateral Mass Fracture

- Mechanism: combined axial loading and lateral bending
- Treatment: stable injury; cervical collar or halo

Jefferson Burst Fracture

- Mechanism: axial loading causing fractures of anterior and posterior parts of the atlas
- Treatment: halo if excursion of lateral masses is greater than 8 mm; otherwise hard collar; if symptomatic nonunion after three months, then occiput to C2 fusion is required

Anterior Arch Fracture

- Mechanism: combined axial load and flexion
- Treatment: hard collar

Transverse Process Fracture

- Mechanism: avulsion injury
- Treatment: usually an incidental finding requiring only symptomatic treatment

Figure 3.6 **C2 (Axis) Dens Fractures (Anderson and D'Alonzo Classification)**

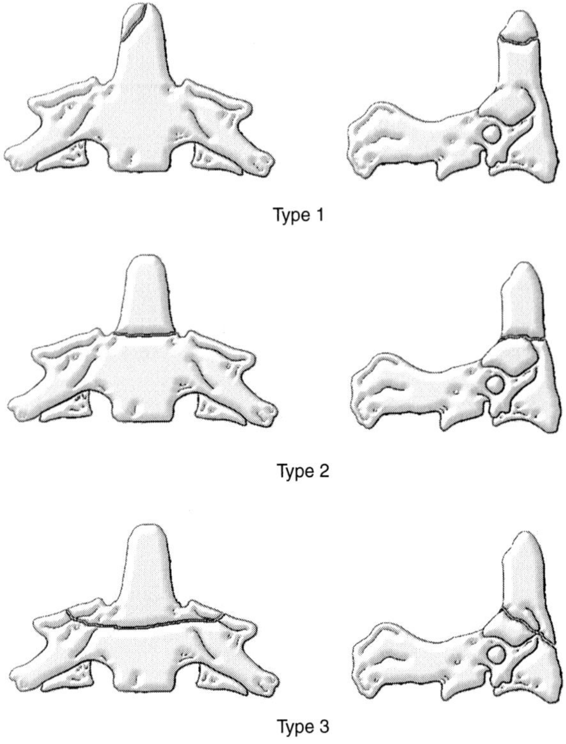

Type 1: oblique fracture through upper part of the dens; treatment is with rigid cervical orthosis such as Philadelphia collar

Type 2: fracture at the junction of the odontoid process and the vertebral body; if displacement is less than 5 mm and angulated less than 15 degrees, then halo is appropriate; otherwise operative treatment with C1 to C2 fusion or screw fixation

Type 3: fracture extends down through vertebral body; treatment is with halo

Figure 3.7 **C2, Posterior Arch or "Hangman's" Fracture (Levine and Edwards Classification)**

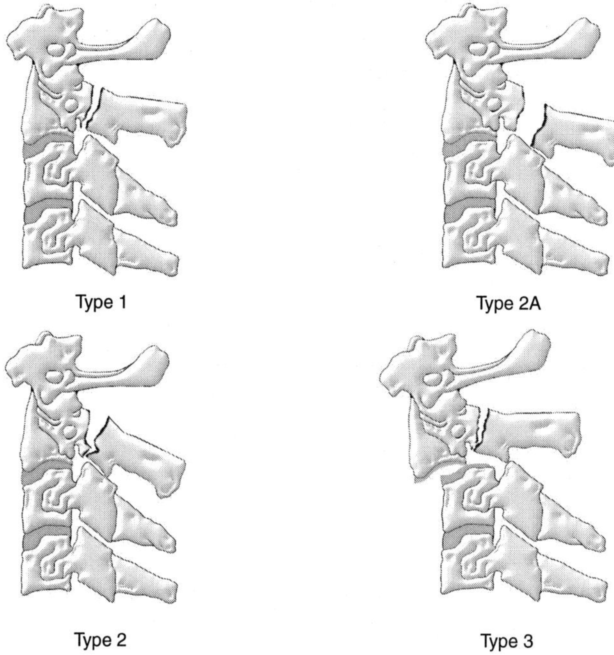

Type 1: fracture with no angulation and less than 3 mm of translation; treatment is with halo

Type 2: fracture with significant angulation and translation (>3 mm); treatment is with halo after closed reduction

Type 2A: fracture with severe angulation but with minimal anterior translation; fragments appear to hinge on the anterior longitudinal ligament; treatment is with halo after closed reduction

Type 3: fracture-dislocation with severe angulation and translation with unilateral or bilateral facet dislocation; treatment is with C1 to C2 fusion

Injuries of the Lower Cervical Spine

There is no clearly accepted classification system. As such, a descriptive system is employed. The basic principles of fracture management apply (i.e., treatment-based stability and presence of neurological deficit).

Spinous Process Fracture (Clay-Shoveler's Fracture)

- Mechanism: flexion injury with avulsion of spinous process; this is a stable injury
- Treatment: requires only symptomatic treatment

Extension Avulsion (Teardrop Fracture)

- Mechanism: hyperextension avulsion of the antero-inferior vertebral body
- Treatment: hard collar

Lamina or Lateral Mass Fracture

- Mechanism: posterior element fracture most often from compressive-extension
- Treatment: hard collar

Facet Dislocation (Unilateral or Bilateral)

- Mechanism: inferior and superior facets are not fractured, however, the superior articular process is anterior to the inferior articular process; this is a flexion distraction injury
- Treatment: if patient is awake, then emergent closed reduction; if patient is not awake, then MRI prior to closed reduction to rule out associated disk herniation; if closed reduction is unsuccessful, then open reduction is necessary

Facet Fracture (Unilateral or Bilateral)

- Mechanism: one of the two articular processes is fractured, with or without a change in the relationship of the inferior to superior facet; this is a flexion compression injury
- Treatment: if patient is awake, then emergent closed reduction; many times, closed reduction is unsuccessful, and open reduction is necessary

Flexion Teardrop

- Mechanism: fracture of the anterior vertebral body from a flexion compression injury
- Treatment: anterior decompression and fusion

Compression Fracture

- Mechanism: axial load injury
- Treatment: hard collar or halo if no instability or malalignment; otherwise anterior interbody fusion

Burst Fracture

- Mechanism: comminuted fracture of vertebral body secondary to axial loading
- Treatment: hard collar or halo if no instability or malalignment; otherwise anterior interbody fusion; if neurologic injury, then anterior decompression prior to fusion

Figure 3.8 **Thoracic and Lumbar Fractures (Orthopedic Trauma Association Classification)**

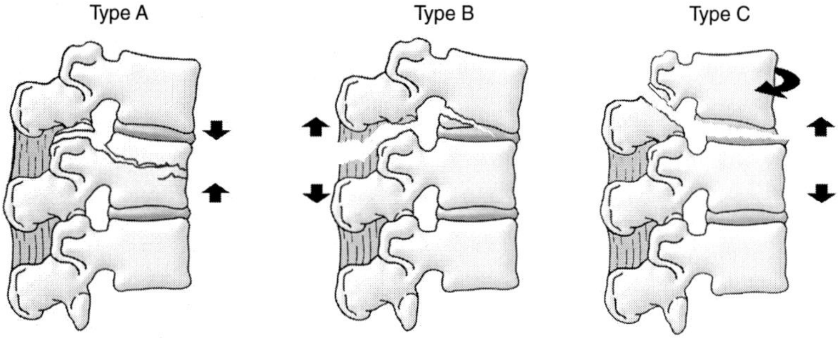

Type A – Vertebral Body Compression

Mechanism: most common injuries caused by axial compression with or without flexion; vertebral body height reduced, but posterior ligamentous complex is intact

Treatment: if stable and no neurological deficit, then brace for three months; if neurological deficit, spine instability or significant deformity is present, then decompression and fusion

Type B – Anterior and Posterior Element Injury with Distraction

Mechanism: fracture with disruption of one or more columns; flexion initiates posterior disruption and elongation, while hyperextension causes anterior disruption and elongation; three subtypes

Treatment: if stable and no neurological deficit, then brace for three months; if neurological deficit is present or spine is unstable, then decompression and fusion

Type C – Anterior and Posterior Element Injury with Rotation

Mechanism: most severe injuries, associated with highest rate of neurological deficit; disruption of all longitudinal ligaments, disks, and articular process fracture; three subtypes

Treatment: fusion, with or without decompression.

Vertical

Fracture line traverses ala, foramen or body of the sacrum

Oblique

May occur at any level and may be associated with concomitant pelvic fracture

Transverse

Least common sacral fracture, but most likely to have neurological deficit

Treatment: most sacral fractures are stable, minimally displaced, and are not associated with neurological deficits; in these cases symptomatic treatment is appropriate (i.e., rest, NSAID, etc.); those injuries associated with neurological deficit require decompression and stabilization; goals of operative management are to reestablish pelvic ring and lumbosacral junction stability, correct and/or prevent angulation or displacement, and prevent neurologic deterioration.

Figure 3.9 **Sacral Fractures**

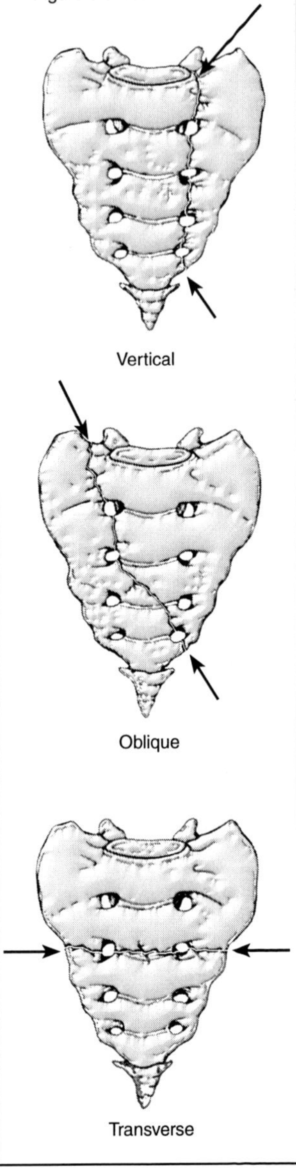

Clinical and Functional Evaluation

Florin Feloiu
Ada Dominguez

Clinicians must incorporate the rehabilitation paradigm into their clinical practice. As such, practitioners must understand the functional consequences of a medical condition. In other words, how does a disorder prevent a patient from performing important life tasks? The activities of daily living (ADL) are the elementary tasks that must be completed for a patient to achieve a basic quality of life. These tasks include dressing, bathing, toileting, feeding, grooming, transfers, ambulating and communicating. The instrumental activities of daily living (IADL) are those essential tasks that allow individuals to interact with the broader community. These tasks include grocery shopping, banking and laundry. Clearly, there is no distinct demarcation between ADL and IADL. Conceptually, ADL and IADL can be performed independently, with modified independence (i.e., with a device), with supervision, or with the assistance of one or even two caregivers.

Once ADL and IADL goals have been reached, patients may pursue vocational and avocational goals. Vocational pursuits may range from unpaid volunteer work (i.e., therapeutic employment) to working with adaptive devices (modified work) to competitive employment. Avocational pursuits include hobbies and recreational activities such as playing chess and water skiing.

Pyramid of Function

Avocational Activities
Vocational Activities
Instrumental Activities of Daily Living
Activities of Daily Living

Levels of Independence

Independent
Modified independence with technology and/or assistive devices
Supervised independence
Assistance of one person
Assistance of two persons

Impairment, Disability and Handicap

Impairment is the lack of normal anatomical or psychological function. Disability is, as the result of an impairment, the inability to perform functional tasks. Handicap is the social disadvantage secondary to a disability. For example, an impairment would be a fractured humerus. As the result of this impairment, the individual requires assistance

in certain ADL, such as dressing and grooming. This individual's handicap is partly determined by his premorbid social, financial and vocational status. If the individual was a psychiatrist, he would essentially have no handicap. On the other hand, if the injured person was a dentist, he would be unable to work and thus would be significantly handicapped.

Measures of Functional Independence

A number of instruments to measure function have been developed, such as the Functional Independence Measure (FIM), Barthel Index, Sister Kenny Index, and Quadriplegia Index of Function. The FIM is the most widely used functional instrument for general rehabilitation units in North America. However, this instrument may not be sensitive or appropriate for functional assessment in spinal cord injury (SCI) patients.

Evaluating SCI Patients

Every SCI patient should be thoroughly evaluated by a physician. This clinical assessment includes a complete physical examination. The International Standards for Neurological Classification of SCI is the most commonly accepted evaluation paradigm. This is commonly known as the ASIA (American Spinal Injury Association) paradigm. Based on the clinical abnormalities ascertained on the International Standards examination, injuries can be categorized utilizing the ASIA Impairment Scale. The ASIA paradigm classifies patients on the basis of their clinical exam, and not by radiological or anatomical abnormalities. The essential elements of the ASIA examination include the bilateral assessment of 10 index muscles (Table 1) and 28 dermatomes. Deep anal pressure (DAP) and voluntary anal sphincteric contraction (VAC) are also evaluated. In addition to the elements of the ASIA examination, a general medical examination, including mental status, cranial nerves and reflexes, should be completed.

The 10 index muscles on each side are evaluated in the supine position. A scale similar to the Medical Research Council Scale is used to grade each index muscle (Table 2). The motor level on each side is at the lowest index muscle with a grade of at least 3, provided that all the index muscles above that level have grade 5 strength. A left and right motor level is obtained, and the patient's motor level is the higher of the two. Table 2 summarizes the assessment of strength for individual index muscles.

Table 1

Key Index Muscles That Must Be Examined

Myotomes	Index Muscle	Action
C5	Biceps Brachialis	Elbow flexors
C6	Extensor Carpi Radialis	Wrist extensors
C7	Triceps	Elbow extensors
C8	Flexor Digitorum Profundus	Finger flexors
T1	Abductor Digiti Minimi	Small finger abductors
L2	Iliopsoas	Hip flexors
L3	Quadriceps	Knee extensors
L4	Tibialis Anterior	Ankle dorsiflexors
L5	Extensor Hallucis Longus	Long toe extensors
S1	Gastrocnemius	Ankle plantarflexors

Table 2
Assessment of Strength

NT	not testable due to immobilization, pain, limb amputation or contracture greater than 50% of the ROM
0	Total Paralysis
1	Palpable or visible contraction
2	Active movement, full ROM with gravity eliminated
3	Active movement, full ROM against gravity
4	Active movement, full ROM against moderate resistance
5	(normal) active movement, full ROM against full resistance expected from an otherwise unimpaired person
5*	(normal) active movement, full ROM against sufficient resistance to be considered normal if identified inhibiting factors were not present

Light touch and pinprick are assessed from 28 dermatomes bilaterally. For every level, a score of 0 (absent), 1 (impaired, which includes partial or altered appreciation), 2 (normal) or NT (not testable) is determined for each modality. Four different sensory scores are generated: left light touch, right light touch, left pinprick, and right pinprick. The sensory score for each side of the body is the sum of the dermatomal sensory scores for both modalities and range from 0 to 112. Based on this clinical assessment, a sensory level can be determined for the left and right sides of the body. The sensory level for one side is defined as the lowest level with entirely normal sensory function (i.e., both pinprick and light touch are normal at and above that level). The patient's sensory level is the higher of the left and right sensory levels.

The digital rectal exam is an essential element of the SCI assessment, as together with the perianal sensory exam, it permits a determination of whether an injury is complete or incomplete. The clinician should insert the index finger into the rectum. Gentle pressure should be applied to the anorectal wall. An alternative technique is to apply pressure to the anus by pressing the thumb, which is outside the rectum, against the index finger, which is inside the rectum. With either technique, DAP is scored as present if the patient consistently appreciates the pressure. Subsequently, the patient should be asked to squeeze down on the examiner's finger to evaluate the presence of volitional contraction of the anal sphincter.

The single neurological level of injury (NLI) is the most caudal segment with normal sensation and antigravity strength on both sides of the body. By definition, the sensory and motor function at all spinal levels above the single NLI have normal sensation (scores of 2 for both light touch and pinprick) and strength (grade 5). Evaluation of the C5 to T1 and L2 to S1 segments involves the assessment of a motor and sensory function. However, all other segments (C2 to C4, T2 to L1 and S2 to S4/5) require only an assessment of sensory function. The single NLI may be assigned based only on the sensory level provided that there is no motor function to be tested at that particular sensory level and, if present, all motor levels above are graded as normal. For example, a patient with a left and right C7 motor level and a left and right C6 sensory level would be assigned a C6 single NLI.

Now consider another case, where an individual had a 5 grade strength in all the index muscles of the upper extremities, a 0 grade strength in the lower extremities, and a left and right T8 sensory level. In this case, the single NLI assigned would be T8.

In summary, four different levels are obtained: left motor, right motor, left sensory and right sensory. On occasion, the process of assigning a single NLI results in misrepresentation of a patient's true impairment. This is particularly evident when there is a marked discrepancy between the motor and sensory levels, or in a lesion with asymmetrical motor and sensory findings. It is advisable to document all four levels, in addition to the single neurological level.

The ASIA Impairment Scale is a modification of the Frankel scale. This paradigm allows for a categorization of an injury as incomplete or complete. An incomplete injury is associated with sacral sparing, which is defined as the presence of some sensation (light touch or pinprick) at the S4-5 dermatome, DAP or VAC on the physical examination. Without any of these three items, the injury is deemed complete. Table 3 summarizes the operational definitions related to the ASIA impairment scale.

The zone of partial preservation (ZPP) is only reported on injuries categorized as complete on the ASIA impairment scale. The ZPP is the most caudal sensory and motor level that remains partially innervated. In the scoring sheet, a ZPP is recorded for both sensory and motor functions on the left and right side of the body.

In this monograph, a standard ASIA exam scoring sheet is attached. The sheet is completed for a hypothetical patient with a C6 neurological level AIS C injury. Table 4 summarizes commonly examined muscle stretch reflexes and the corresponding nerve roots.

Table 3
ASIA Impairment Scale

A	**Complete:** No motor or sensory function is preserved in the sacral segments S4–S5.
B	**Sensory Incomplete:** Sensory but not motor function is preserved below the neurological level and includes the sacral segments S4–S5, and no motor function is preserved more than 3 levels below the motor level on either side of the body.
C	**Motor incomplete:** Motor function is preserved below the neurological level, and more than half of key muscles below the neurological level have a muscle grade less than 3.
D	**Motor incomplete:** Motor function is preserved below the neurological level, and at least half of key muscles below the neurological level have a muscle grade of greater than or equal to 3.
E	**Normal:** Motor and sensory function are normal.

Note: When assessing the extent of motor sparing below the level for distinguishing between B and C, the motor level on each side is used. To differentiate between C and D the single neurological level is used.

Patient Name Hypot

Examiner Name Jan

AMERICAN SPINAL INJURY ASSOCIATION

	R	L	
C5	5	5	Elbo
C6	5	5	Wris
C7	5	2	Elbo
C8	5	0	Fing
T1	4	1	Fing
UPPER LIMB TOTAL (MAXIMUM)	24 (25)	+ 13 (25)	=

Comments:

Right Hamstring

Lt Hamstring 0/5

Rt Hip Adductors

Lt Hip Adductors

L2	0	1	Hip fle
L3	0	0	Knee
L4	3	2	Ankle
L5	2	2	Long t
S1	0	0	Ankle

(VAC) Vol

LOWER LIMB TOTAL (MAXIMUM): 5 (25) + 5 (25) = 1 (50)

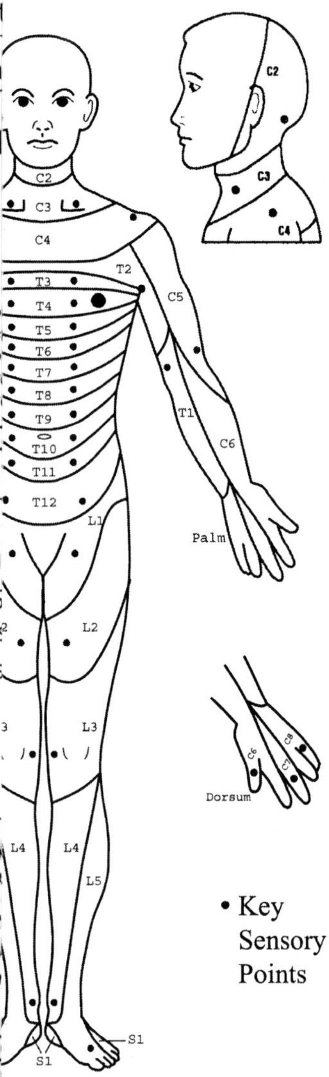

NEUROLOGICAL LEVEL
The most caudal segment with normal function

SENS
MOT

juries only)
PARTIAL ...**VATION**
...al level ...nervation

	R	L
SENSORY	NA	NA
MOTOR	NA	NA

This

Steps in Evaluating an SCI Patient

1. Examine 10 index muscles bilaterally
2. Examine 28 dermatomes bilaterally for pinprick and light touch
3. Complete rectal exam to assess deep anal pressure and voluntary contraction of anal sphincter
4. Determine left and right sensory levels
5. Determine left and right motor levels
6. Assign "final" motor and sensory levels
7. Determine the single neurological level of injury
8. Categorize injury as complete or incomplete by ASIA impairment scale (A, B, C, D, E)
9. Calculate motor and sensory score
10. Determine zone of partial preservation if complete injury ("A" on impairment scale)

Table 4
Muscle Stretch Reflexes and Corresponding Nerve Roots

Stretch Reflex	Predominant Motor/Root Level
Biceps	C5
Brachioradialis	C6
Triceps	C7
Finger Flexor	C8
Quadriceps	L4
Hamstrings	L5
Gastrocnemius	S1

Discrepancy Between Anatomical and ASIA Neurological Level of Injury

Many times, there is a discrepancy between the anatomical level of injury (the level with the greatest anatomical injury found on imaging modalities) and the neurological level of injury. For example, a patient with a C6 burst fracture may have sparing of the C7 motor level. This is because the motor neuron pool for any myotome is cephalad to the corresponding vertebral body. As a guideline, the motor neuron pool is one segment cephalad to the corresponding vertebral body in the cervical spine, two segments higher in the thoracic spine, and three segments higher in the lumbar spine.

Complete vs. Incomplete Injury

Complete injuries imply absent sensation to light touch and pinprick in the S4-5 dermatomal area, absent DAP and VAC. The AIS provides operational definitions of the terms complete and incomplete; however, most patients (and some clinicians) do not characterize injuries on the basis of the most recent AIS criterion. Of note, most patients with spinal cord injury do not have total anatomical severance of the spinal cord. This phenomenon is sometimes categorized as "discomplete." On occasion, these terms can be a source of confusion.

Upper and Lower Motor Neuron Injury

It is important to understand the concept of upper and lower motor neuron injury. Volitional movement of muscle groups requires an intact upper and lower motor neuron supply. The upper motor neuron supply (i.e., corticospinal tract) begins in the prefrontal motor cortex, travels through the internal capsule and brain stem, and projects into the spinal cord. The lower motor neuron supply begins in the anterior horn cells of the spinal cord and includes the peripheral nerves. Most lesions in the cervical and thoracic cord result in predominantly upper motor neuron injury. However, at the level of the injury, there may be limited lower motor neuron injury with compromise of the nerve roots and/or the anterior horn cells. Upper motor neuron lesions are associated with upper motor neuron findings such as increased muscle stretch reflexes, clonus, Babinski (extensor) response, and detrusor sphincter dyssynergia. The terminal segment of the spinal cord, the conus medullaris, is located at approximately the L1 to L2 vertebral body. Injuries below the L2 vertebral body (below the conus medullaris of the spinal cord) result in lower motor neuron injury. Lower motor neuron lesions are characterized by hyporeflexia, flaccid weakness, and significant muscle wasting. Lesions at the upper lumbar vertebral bodies can present with a mixture of upper and lower motor neuron findings due to injury of the conus medullaris.

Spinal Shock

It is sometimes difficult to clinically distinguish between upper and lower motor neuron injury immediately after SCI due to "spinal shock." Spinal shock is a commonly used term that refers to the lack of descending facilitation after an upper motor neuron lesion. The patient will initially have findings consistent with lower motor neuron injury, with upper motor neuron findings typically developing over a period of days to weeks.

Chapter 5

Functional Outcomes by Level of Injury

Shanker Nesathurai

Patients, families and clinicians may inquire about an individual's ultimate functional capability after completing a rehabilitation program. Physicians must be able to provide cautious, but realistic advice. The following is a general discussion of functional capability by motor level. Although not the exclusive determinant, functional independence is closely correlated with motor level.

With the exception of a complete anatomical spinal cord transection, it is difficult to predict with confidence on the ultimate return of strength distal to the neurological level. It is not unusual for individuals to gain one motor level over the first year of injury. Some patients with apparently devastating injuries regain significant strength distal to their level of injury; others make no recovery whatsoever.

C2 to C4 Tetraplegia

Patients with C2 to C4 lesions are the most profoundly injured SCI patients and are commonly referred to as "high tetraplegics." These patients have no significant strength in any limb. Many are ventilator dependent and have long-term tracheostomies. These patients require assistance for all ADL and IADL. A caregiver must be available on a 24-hour basis. Mobility requires a power wheelchair. Intermittent catheterization is ideal, but an attendant must be available to perform this procedure four to six times per day. As a practical matter, most high tetraplegics have an indwelling urinary catheter (Foley or suprapubic).

Technological advances have clearly improved the quality of these patients' lives. A ventilator dependent patient may require a "talking" tracheostomy to communicate. Computer-driven environmental control systems that interface with voice, sip-and-puff, or chin control mechanisms allow patients to perform tasks such as turning on lights or opening a door.

The phrenic nerve supplies the diaphragm and is supplied by the C3, C4, and C5 motor neuron pool. On occasion, electrical stimulation of the phrenic nerve or diaphragm can liberate a high tetraplegic from the ventilator for at least part of the day. The lower motor neuron pathways must be intact to pace the phrenic nerve. Nerve conduction studies of the phrenic nerve and an EMG of the diaphragm can help determine if pacing is a viable option.

C5 Tetraplegia

Patients with this motor level have some preserved biceps function. These individuals should be able to assist in their self-care activities (e.g., grooming, bathing and toileting). C5 tetraplegics will require adaptive devices to feed independently (e.g., universal cuffs). C5 tetraplegics cannot perform intermittent self-catheterization. As a practical matter, bladder management will require an indwelling catheter. C5 tetraplegics will require assistance for transfers. Mobility will be with a power wheelchair.

centers. The bladder is innervated by sympathetic (T10 to L2, hypogastric nerve), parasympathetic (S2 to S4, pelvic nerve), and somatic (S2 to S4, pudendal nerve) fibers. If the injury affects the peripheral innervation of the bladder or completely destroys the conus medullaris, lower motor neuron bladder dysfunction may be present. If the lesion is above the sacral micturition center, the result will be an upper motor neuron bladder.

With lower motor neuron bladder dysfunction, sphincter and/or bladder tone may be absent or diminished. Patients may experience urinary incontinence or the inability to void. In the acute phase of injury, the clinical abnormalities of upper and lower motor neuron bladder dysfunction will be similar. In injuries above the sacral micturition center, the classical findings of an upper motor neuron bladder may become apparent when spinal shock resolves. Upper motor neuron bladder pathology is characterized by low urinary volumes, high bladder pressures, and uninhibited detrusor contractions. Detrusor sphincter dyssynergia (DSD) is common in lesions between the sacral and pontine micturition centers. DSD is characterized by co-contraction of the bladder and urinary sphincter. Untreated, upper motor neuron bladder dysfunction can lead to incontinence, vesicoureteral reflux, and hydronephrosis.

Most acutely injured patients will have a Foley catheter. When the patient is stable, and total urinary output is less than 2,000 cc, an intermittent catheterization program (ICP) should be started. Initially, the ICP should be on a q4 hour basis, with target volumes between 400 cc to 500 cc. If volumes are consistently small, the frequency of catheterization can be increased to q6h. The bladder management program can be individualized during the rehabilitation phase of care. Some SCI patients may be able to manage bladder dysfunction by other methods, including the Valsalva maneuver, manual suprapubic pressure (Crede maneuver), suprapubic tapping, or a condom catheter. Please refer to chapter 7 for a more detailed discussion.

Bowel Management

Most patients with upper motor neuron pathology (lesions above the conus medullaris) will likely suffer from constipation. In lower motor neuron pathology, fecal incontinence is possible during acute hospitalization, although most of these patients will experience constipation in the post-acute phase. Opioids and tricyclic agents may exacerbate constipation. A comprehensive bowel regimen should be instituted. In an acute injury, stool softeners, such as ducusate (Colace) or senna preparations (Senokot), can be started. The patient should be placed on the commode after breakfast to utilize the gastrocolic reflex. If obstipation is suspected, a KUB film should be obtained and a gentle enema can be considered.

Abdominal distention, pancreatitis, and gastric ulcers are possible in the acute phase of injury. The patient should be encouraged to eat when the paralytic ileus resolves. Please refer to chapter 8 for a more detailed discussion.

Pressure Ulcers

Pressure ulcers are an avoidable complication in SCI patients. The amount of time a vulnerable area is subjected to pressure should be minimized. Excessive shear forces and moisture should also be avoided. The development of an ulcer can profoundly impact the nature and length of a patient's rehabilitation care. The best way to prevent pressure ulcers is to turn and position the patient every two hours. Clinicians should monitor the

skin closely. Extreme care must be used in assisted bed mobility and transfers. Maceration of the skin by urine, feces and excessive perspiration can contribute to ulcers. If there are areas of threatened skin breakdown, an alternative bed surface should be considered. Please refer to chapter 9 for a more detailed discussion.

Contractures

Immobility leads to contractures, and can be prevented. Muscles that cross two joints, such as the gastrocnemius, hamstrings, iliopsoas and biceps brachii, are at particular risk. Contractures can be prevented by passive range of movement of the joints and proper positioning (e.g., prone lying to minimize iliopsoas contractures). The physical therapy service can assist in contracture prevention. An ankle foot orthosis can prevent the progression of gastrocnemius contractures. However, an orthosis is not a substitute for a passive range of movement program. In a minority of cases, contractures should be encouraged. For example, in a patient with C6 tetraplegia, the MCP, PIP and DIP joints should be allowed to contract in approximately 20 degrees of flexion. These contractures will assist in providing a functional grasp. A volar wrist hand orthosis can help facilitate this beneficial contracture. If the spine has not been stabilized, the passive range of movement program must be approved by the surgeons to minimize any further potential spinal cord compromise. Please refer to chapter 10 for a more detailed discussion.

Autonomic Dysfunction

Patients with SCI commonly suffer from dysautonomia. In the acute phase (during spinal shock), patients may experience orthostatic hypotension, tachycardia or bradycardia. Orthostatic hypotension can be minimized by slowly elevating a patient's head and cautiously allowing the patient's legs to hang over the edge of the bed. Thigh high compression stockings and an abdominal binder can be helpful. Fludrocortisone acetate (Florinef) and ephedrine can also be used in refractory cases. Some patients will suffer from bradycardia with pulmonary suctioning due to increased vagal stimulation. In these cases, pretreatment with atropine (1 mg intravenously) and/or preoxygenation can be useful.

Disorders of temperature regulation are common in tetraplegic patients. "Quad fevers" are when SCI patients have high temperatures (i.e., above 104 degrees Fahrenheit), but have no other findings consistent with infection. These patients "look well," although they have very high body temperatures. This diagnosis should only be made when all other causes of fever have been reasonably excluded. Patients may also experience poikilothermia in which body temperature is affected by ambient temperature. Adjusting the thermostat can resolve this problem.

Autonomic dysreflexia (AD) is a syndrome characterized by headache, flushing, piloerection, hypertension and tachycardia. It is not commonly encountered in the first few weeks of SCI, but rather when a patient emerges from spinal shock. Patients with lesions above T6 are at greatest risk, although there are reports of AD with lesions below this level. **This condition is an emergency and requires immediate intervention.** If untreated, autonomic dysreflexia can lead to stroke, seizures and even death. Any noxious stimulus below the level of injury can precipitate AD. Common causes of AD include bladder distention or fecal impaction. Less common causes include pressure ulcers, ingrown toe nails, nephrolithiasis, tight clothing or heterotopic ossification.

Acute abdominal pathology, such as cholecystitis or perforated viscus, can also cause autonomic dysreflexia. The initial management of AD includes elevating the head. If possible, the patient's legs should be allowed to hang from the bed in order to decrease venous return. The precipitating cause must be identified and treated. If the etiology cannot be ascertained promptly, the hypertension must be treated. A variety of agents are available, including topical nitrates, calcium channel blockers, beta blockers and centrally acting alpha agonists. Please refer to chapter 11 for a more detailed discussion.

Upper Motor Neuron Syndrome and Spasticity

Spasticity is a disorder of muscle tone characterized by a velocity dependent resistance to passive joint movement. Other manifestations of spasticity include increased muscle stretch reflexes, clonus and the "clasp-knife" phenomenon. Flexor and cutaneo-motor spasms are common in upper motor neuron diseases. Although these abnormalities are not considered manifestations of spasticity, they may cause significant functional limitation. Spasms can be treated with many of the same management strategies as spasticity. Spasticity becomes more apparent as a patient emerges from spinal shock. Spasticity may be treated when it contributes to pain, impairs hygiene, interferes with nursing care, contributes to contractures, or leads to pressure ulcers. However, some patients find spasticity helpful with mobility and transfers. As such, the risks and benefits of intervention should be balanced.

Chronic SCI patients who are admitted to the hospital should remain on their spasticity medications. This is particularly important in patients who are on baclofen, as rapid withdrawal can lead to seizures, weakness and mental status changes.

Spasticity can be managed with medications such as baclofen (Lioresal), tizanidine (Zanaflex), diazepam (Valium), dantrolene sodium (Dantrium), and clonidine (Catapres). Other interventions include motor branch blocks, nerve blocks and botulinum toxin injections. In refractory cases, an intrathecal baclofen pump can be considered. Please refer to chapter 12 for a more detailed discussion.

Venous Thromboembolism Prophylaxis

SCI patients are at very high risk for developing deep venous thrombosis (DVT). As DVT can lead to pulmonary emboli and potentially death, prophylaxis is essential. The therapeutic options include intermittent pneumatic compression devices (e.g., Venodyne boots), thigh high graded compression stockings (e.g., TED stockings), warfarin, minidose subcutaneous unfractionated heparin (5,000 units bid), adjusted dose subcutaneous unfractionated heparin, or low molecular weight heparin (LMWH). A Greenfield filter also may be indicated in selected cases. Low molecular weight heparin is probably the best choice to prevent VTE. There are many LMWH products commercially available, including enoxaparin, dalteparin, nadroparin, troparin and bemiparin. However, some surgeons and critical care physicians are concerned about potential bleeding in the spinal cord and are hesitant to start anticoagulants in the acute phase of injury. When there are strong reservations about low molecular weight heparin, utilization of intermittent compression devices and compression stockings in addition to serial doppler surveillance may be a reasonable compromise. However, serial doppler studies are expensive and fail to detect a significant number of calf thrombosis. In high risk patients (i.e., complete high quadriplegia with femur fracture) where LMWH cannot be prescribed, a Greenfield

filter may be considered. Later, in the rehabilitation phase of management, low molecular weight heparin can be instituted.

Pulmonary Management

Normal ventilation requires the diaphragm (C3 to C5), intercostal (T1 to T12), upper abdominal muscles (T8 to T10), and lower abdominal muscles (T10 to T12). Tetraplegics may have paralysis of the intercostal and abdominal muscles. In tetraplegia, the accessory muscles of ventilation, such as scalene anticus, scalene medius, levator scapula and trapezius, are usually spared. These muscles are essential for ventilation. Intercostal and abdominal muscle weakness results in an impaired cough and subsequent difficulty clearing secretions. Pneumonia is commonly encountered. Aggressive chest physical therapy techniques, such as assisted cough ("quad cough"), chest wall percussion, breath stacking, and postural draining positioning, may decrease secretions and mucus plugging.

High tetraplegics (i.e., those with lesions above C4) many times are unable to be weaned off the ventilator. These patients will require tracheostomy and long-term ventilation. High tetraplegics who have some intact lower motor neuron supply to the diaphragm may benefit from electrical stimulation of the phrenic nerve or diaphragm. With this intervention, some high tetraplegics may be liberated from a ventilator for some part of the day.

Psychological Adaptation

Patients with catastrophic SCI may experience a range of emotions, including denial, anger, guilt, disbelief and frustration. There is no "normal" pattern of coping. Families also may require emotional and psychological support. The rehabilitation psychology, social work and pastoral care services may provide comfort and support. These services should be consulted early in SCI. Please refer to chapter 14 for a more detailed discussion.

Pain

Patients with acute lesions can experience significant pain. Pain should be treated with judicious use of opioid and non-opioid analgesics. Many patients complain of neuropathic pain which may be manifested by poorly localized dysesthesias. This can be treated with low dose tricyclic agents, such as amitriptyline (Elavil), nortriptyline (Pamelor), or imipramine (Tofranil). These agents have anticholinergic side effects such as dry mouth, light headedness, blurred vision, and orthostatic hypotension. Carbamazepine (Tegretol), gabapentin (Neurontin), phenytoin (Dilantin) and pregablin (Lyrica) may also palliate neuropathic pain. Non-pharmacological interventions to control pain include transcutaneous electrical nerve stimulation (TENS) and acupuncture. Psychological pain management techniques can be considered, including hypnosis and relaxation therapy.

In chronic spinal cord patients who are admitted for concurrent surgical procedures, adequate pain relief is essential. Autonomic dysreflexia and increased spasticity can be precipitated by untreated pain.

Hypercalcemia

After a spinal cord injury, there is an efflux of calcium from bones below the level of the injury, also known as immobilization hypercalcemia. This is more common in young men with SCI. If unmanaged, patients may experience fatigue, lethargy, nausea, and even

psychosis. Other features include vomiting, abdominal pain, polydipsia, dehydration, renal failure, and nephrolithiasis. Intravenous normal saline is an appropriate first-line treatment. Other treatments include biphosphonates and loop diuretics. In severe cases, calcitonin can be prescribed.

Comorbid Conditions

Many persons with SCI have other injuries such as fractures, abdominal wounds, traumatic brain injuries, seizure disorders, pneumothorax, cardiac contusions, and peripheral nerve injuries. Some patients also have substance abuse disorders. These co-existing impairments must be documented in the consultation record. Comorbid conditions could affect the rehabilitation care a patient requires. For example, a patient with an L5 paraplegia should be able to walk with braces. However, if the injured individual also has an acetabular fracture, he may not be permitted to bear weight for many weeks. As such, wheelchair-level goals would be appropriate for this patient.

SCI can be associated with concomitant head injuries. Sometimes, traumatic brain injuries (TBI) are unrecognized due to relative subtle deficits or normal neuroimaging. A negative CT scan or MRI of the brain, however, does not exclude a traumatic brain injury. A mental status exam should be completed whenever possible. If there is a high index of suspicion, a neuropsychological consultation should be obtained.

Patients with TBI and SCI present a unique challenge to the rehabilitation team. The team will have to manage the sequelae of TBI (agitation, memory impairments, attention deficits) in addition to SCI issues. More resources will be required to achieve equal functional gains in an SCI patient with concomitant TBI.

Disposition and Discharge Planning

Discharge planning should begin as soon as the patient is admitted to the hospital. Physiatrists should advocate for appropriate comprehensive spinal cord injury care. Institutions with SCI programs certified by the Commission on the Accreditation of Rehabilitation Facilities (CARF) or designated as National Model Spinal Cord Injury System Centers will probably provide excellent care. Insurance carriers may compel patients to receive rehabilitation services from "preferred" providers. Some patients will request rehabilitation services at sites close to their homes or for other personal reasons.

Community Reintegration

During the initial in-hospital consultation, it is important to comment on the community reintegration plan. This plan includes identifying a primary care physician and physiatrist with expertise in SCI. Patients should be encouraged to participate in routine health maintenance activities such as regular immunizations and screening for colon cancer and cardiovascular disease. The long-term issues related to SCI are discussed in more detail in chapter 19 and 20.

Checklist for Acute Spinal Cord Injury Rehabilitation Medicine Consultation

- Detailed Clinical Summary of Injury
- Document Comorbid Conditions
- Comprehensive Physical Examination
- Document ASIA Assessment

Comment on the Following Issues

- Bladder
- Bowel
- Pressure Ulcers
- Contracture Prevention
- Dysautonomia
- Spasticity
- Psychological Adaptation
- DVT Prophylaxis
- Pulmonary
- Pain
- Comorbid Conditions
- Disposition and Discharge Planning
- Community Reintegration

Chapter 7

Bladder Management

Shanker Nesathurai
Dinesh Kumbhare

Introduction

The mortality and morbidity associated with urological disease is significant in the SCI population. After World War II, renal failure was the leading cause of death in persons with SCI. With advances in urological management, renal disease is now the fourth leading cause of death.

The two major functions of the bladder are storage and emptying of urine. This complex activity requires the coordinated function of the peripheral nervous system, sacral micturition center, pontine micturition center, and the cerebral cortex. In infants, voiding is not meaningfully influenced by the cortex, and voiding is initiated reflexively in response to bladder fullness. In adults, the pontine micturition center is modulated by higher centers, which facilitate voiding at socially appropriate times.

Innervation of the Lower Urinary Tract

The lower urinary tract is innervated by the somatic, parasympathetic and sympathetic nervous systems. The somatic nuclei are located in the anterior horn of the gray matter of the S2 to S4 spinal cord. These fibers project through the pudendal nerve to innervate the external urethral sphincter (striated muscle). In the absence of an SCI, the external sphincter is under voluntary control. Preganglionic parasympathetic neurons originate in the intermediolateral horn of the gray matter of the S2 to S4 segments. These fibers travel through the pelvic nerves to the prostatic plexus. Postganglionic parasympathetic fibers originating in the prostatic plexus then supply the detrusor of the bladder. Stimulation of the parasympathetic fibers will facilitate detrusor contraction and voiding. The sympathetic (alpha and beta adrenergic) fibers originate in the T10 to L2 spinal segments and project through the sympathetic chain and inferior mesenteric ganglion. These neurons travel to the bladder via the hypogastric nerve. The alpha adrenergic sympathetic neurons supply the bladder neck (internal sphincter). The stimulation of alpha adrenergic nerves will cause contraction of the bladder neck; this is the primary mechanism that promotes urinary continence and prevents retrograde ejaculation. Beta adrenergic stimulation will inhibit detrusor contraction and assist in urinary storage. Research also suggests that afferent A-delta and C fibers are also involved in physiological voiding.

Spinal Tracts Affecting Bladder Function

Sensory impulses from the proprioceptive nerve endings in the mucosal wall of the bladder, abdominal wall, urethra and periurethral areas travel through the lateral

somatic and posterior columns in the spinal cord. These impulses are relayed to different areas of the brain. Motor control of bladder and sphincter function is modulated by the descending bulbospinal, reticulospinal and cerulospinal tracts.

Coordination of Micturition

The pontine micturition center coordinates contraction and relaxation of the detrusor and sphincter. During urination, the detrusor muscle contracts after the sphincter relaxes. During storage, the opposite must occur; the detrusor muscle must relax while the sphincter contracts (guarding reflex). This coordination of the contraction and relaxation is called detrusor sphincter synergia.

The medial frontal lobe, corpus callosum, limbic system, hypothalamus, basal ganglia and cerebellum are all involved in the control of bladder function. They exert either facilitatory or inhibitory influences upon the bladder by projecting impulses through the pontine micturition center or directly to the sacral segments.

Medical and Social Issues Related to SCI Bladder Management

Clinicians must be sensitive to both the medical and social issues related to SCI bladder dysfunction. From a medical perspective, the primary goal is to preserve renal function. Repeated upper urinary tract infections and vesicoureteral reflux will contribute to renal scarring and progressive renal failure. In addition, urinary incontinence can cause skin maceration, which can contribute to skin breakdown.

Bladder dysfunction has significant social consequences. Frequently, the injured person will have urinary incontinence. Some patients may have to rely on others for catheterization or for the cleaning of soiled bed linens and clothing. This may result in personal embarrassment. These feelings can be compounded if family members must perform these tasks.

Lower Motor Neuron Bladder Dysfunction

Bladder dysfunction is closely related to the level of the injury. If the lesion involves the peripheral innervation of the bladder or destroys the sacral micturition center, the result is a lower motor neuron bladder. This type of bladder pathology may be associated with a hypotonic detrusor and/or sphincter. Consequently, clinical findings may include urinary retention with associated overflow incontinence. Alternatively, incontinence may be secondary to diminished sphincter tone.

Upper Motor Neuron Bladder Dysfunction and Detrusor Sphincter Dyssynergia

If the SCI is above the sacral micturition center, the result is an upper motor neuron bladder; this type of dysfunction is characterized by low urinary volumes, high bladder pressures, bladder trabeculation, and diminished bladder compliance. In some cases, uninhibited detrusor contractions ("bladder spasms") may trigger autonomic dysreflexia. Most patients with upper motor neuron bladders will have some incontinence. Many patients (perhaps more than 90 percent) with SCI develop detrusor sphincter dyssynergia (DSD). This condition is common in neurological injuries between the sacral and pontine micturition center. DSD is characterized by co-contraction of the bladder and sphincter.

Vesicoureteral Reflux

The distal portion of the ureter enters into the bladder at an oblique angle, and the ureteral meatus opens at the posterolateral portion of the trigone. Increased intravesical pressure will usually compress the submucosal portion of the ureter against the detrusor muscle, thus obliterating the ureter. Because of this valve mechanism, vesicoureteral reflux (VUR) is absent in healthy adults. The effectiveness of this valve mechanism depends on the ratio of ureteral diameter to the length of the submucosal ureter.

The bladder is able to eliminate urine only when the intravesical pressure exceeds the urethral pressure. Therefore, voiding may be incomplete with DSD. The urine remaining in the bladder is the post void residual (PVR) volume. High PVR (perhaps greater than 100 cc) with elevated intravesical pressures may be associated with vesicoureteral reflux. In this case, with bladder contraction, some of the urine travels through the incompetent ureter-bladder valve mechanism and into the kidneys.

There is no consensus on absolute intravesical pressure that will lead to VUR. Intravesical pressures of 40 cm to 60 cm of water may be associated with VUR. The diagnosis of VUR may be confirmed by a voiding cystogram.

Urodynamic Studies

Urodynamic studies (Figure 7.1) are important in assessing the nature of voiding function. However, this study must be utilized in conjunction with good clinical judgment and may have some limitations. Urodynamic findings may change from the acute phase of injury to the chronic phase. This is especially true in upper motor neuron and mixed lesions. Arguably, some components of this test do not mimic physiological bladder function. For example, in some labs the bladder is filled with gas at a rapid rate. With physiological urological function, the bladder is filled slowly through the ureters with fluid. Psychological stress can also affect urodynamic findings, especially the initiation of voiding. In addition, a urodynamic study is a sample of a single storage-voiding cycle and may not be representative of the bladder being tested. Finally, the results can be affected by the instrumentation, type of catheter used, and the position of the patient during testing.

Management of Lower Motor Neuron Bladder Dysfunction

This type of bladder pathology will result in two possible clinical scenarios. In the first scenario, sphincter tone is diminished; however, detrusor tone is normal or compromised. This individual will have continuous incontinence. For a male patient, a condom catheter will be satisfactory. In a female patient, an indwelling catheter will be required. Theoretically, sphincter tone can be increased with alpha adrenergic medications (i.e., ephedrine). However, as a practical matter, this is unlikely to result in socially acceptable continence. In selected cases, an artificial sphincter may permit continence. The second scenario is where the sphincter is competent to maintain acceptable continence, but bladder tone is diminished and the individual cannot micturate. In this scenario, an intermittent catheterization program (ICP) can be recommended. Another alternative is bladder evacuation with the Valsalva maneuver or suprapubic pressure (Crede maneuver).

Figure 7.1 **Typical Urodynamic Study**

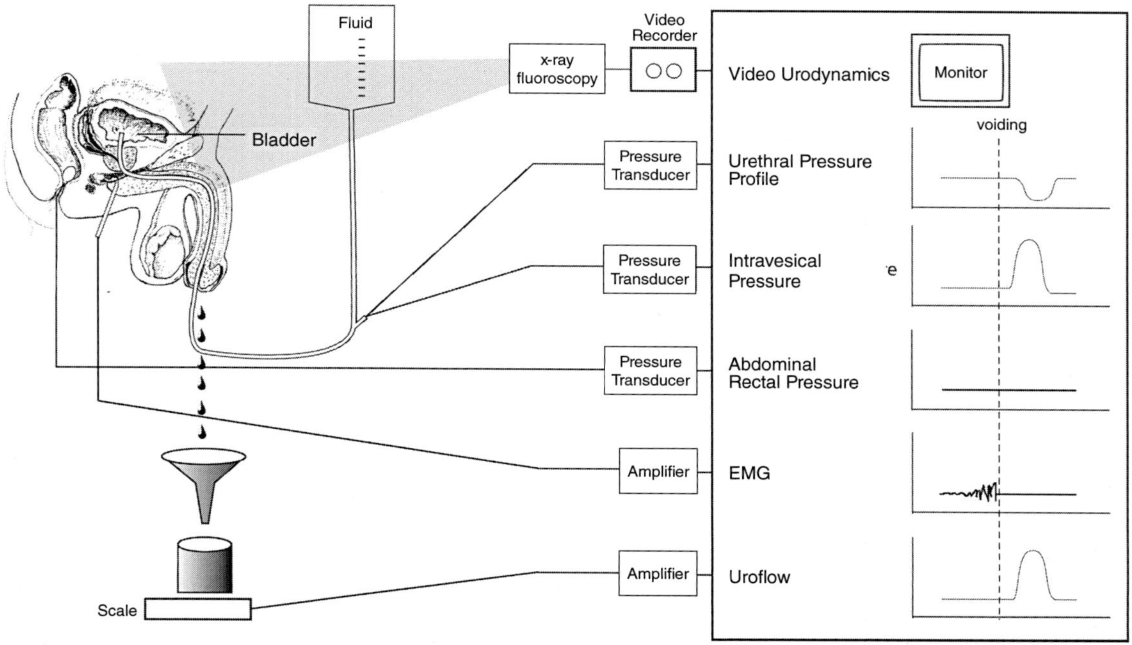

Instrumentation for urodynamic studies is not standardized. The illustration above uses radio-opaque fluid. Some physicians, however, prefer to use carbon dioxide. Normal bladder function can be divided into storage and voiding phases. The first sensation of bladder filling is between 100 cc and 200 cc. The patient experiences bladder fullness between 300 cc and 400 cc and the sense of urgency between 400 cc and 500 cc. Intravesical pressure does not increase significantly during the storage phase due to the vesicoelasticity of the vesical wall. During the voiding phase, sphincter activity stops and the bladder contracts. During normal voiding, the EMG signal will be silent, intravesical pressure will increase, and urethral pressure will decrease. Fluoroscopy will qualitatively assess bladder contraction and document any potential vesicoureteral reflux.

Both of these maneuvers are associated with incomplete bladder emptying, increased vesicoureteral reflux and possible hernia, pelvic organ prolapse and hemorrhoids. This strategy should be avoided in the presence of significant detrusor sphincter dyssynergia or bladder outlet obstruction. An indwelling catheter is a less satisfactory treatment for this type of bladder dysfunction. Cholinergic agonists such as bethanechol chloride (Urecholine) are ineffective in increasing detrusor tone in SCI.

Management of Upper Motor Neuron Bladder Dysfunction

During spinal shock, patients with upper motor neuron and lower motor neuron bladder dysfunction will have similar clinical abnormalities. Consequently, the management strategies will be similar.

As spinal shock resolves, the manifestations of an upper motor neuron bladder will become evident. Most patients with upper motor neuron bladder dysfunction will have some incontinence. At this stage, a urodynamic study will assist in clarifying the nature of voiding function.

Medications with anticholinergic properties such as oxybutynin, imipramine, propantheline bromide will decrease detrusor tone and allow for greater bladder capacity (Table 1). This intervention may also reduce VUR and uninhibited bladder contractions. SCI patients with upper motor neuron bladder dysfunction who are able to engage in an ICP may benefit from these medications. As well, a few persons with incomplete or mixed lesions may utilize suprapubic tapping in conjunction with anticholinergic medications.

On rare occasions, bladder augmentation can increase bladder capacity. This is a surgical procedure that increases vesical volume by interposing a piece of small bowel with bladder tissue. The patient can then engage in an ICP. A competent sphincter is required for this bladder management strategy.

Patients who have upper motor neuron bladders and are unable to use an ICP will require an indwelling catheter (preferably a suprapubic catheter). In male patients, an alternative management strategy could be a transurethral sphincterotomy or transurethral stent, which would lead to continuous incontinence. A condom catheter could then be employed.

Micturition requires detrusor pressures to exceed bladder outlet pressures. Some individuals with SCI may not be able to void as a result of increased internal sphincter tone. Medications and procedures may successfully decrease outlet obstruction and thereby allow voiding with suprapubic tapping, Valsalva maneuver or manual suprapubic pressure (Crede maneuver). Alpha adrenergic antagonists, such as terazosin, prazosin, doxazosin or tamsulosin, may decrease internal sphincter tone (Table 2). However, these medications may cause significant hypotension, and the doses should be carefully titrated. In men, a sphincterotomy which moderately decreases outlet obstruction may improve bladder emptying. However, many patients are rendered incontinent and will require a condom catheter. Other side effects include bleeding and loss of erectile function. Recurrence of urinary obstruction may occur due to fibrosis and subsequent procedures may be required. In male patients, external sphincter tone can be decreased with transurethral or transperineal botulinum toxin. This procedure is not recommended in women as it may result in incontinence. The effects of botulinum toxin range from three to six months. To decrease external sphincter tone (striated muscle), baclofen, diazepam and dantrolene may be considered; however, these medications are usually unsuccessful.

Table 1
Medications With Anticholinergic Properties That Decrease Bladder Tone

Medication	Brand Name	Initial Dose	Maximum Dose	Precautions
oxybutynin chloride	Ditropan	5 mg bid	5 mg qid	dry mouth blurred vision rash nausea vomiting sedation tachycardia urinary retention constipation
imipramine hcl	Tofranil	10 mg tid	50 mg tid	dry mouth blurred vision sedation tachycardia nausea vomiting orthostatic hypotension photosensitivity
propantheline bromide	Pro-Banthine	7.5 mg tid	30 mg tid and qhs	dry mouth blurred vision palpitations headache sedation

Guidelines for an Intermittent Catheterization Program

Many times, an intermittent catheterization program (ICP) is the preferred method of treating bladder dysfunction. An ICP may be started when the patient is medically stable and daily urine output is less than 2,000 cc. ICP should be initiated at four- or six-hour intervals. Acceptable catheterization volumes should not exceed 400 cc to 500 cc. Larger amounts may result in bladder distention and excessive intravesical pressure. The primary method of regulating urinary output is fluid intake. Persons with SCI should be encouraged to adjust fluid consumption accordingly in order to minimize excessive catheterization volumes. A detailed diary of fluid intake and catheter volumes should be maintained.

A four-times-a-day ICP is more practical than a strict every-six-hour program; a strict every-six-hour program would require waking the person with SCI during the night. In addition, those individuals who cannot perform self-catheterization may have difficulty finding a caregiver to perform intermittent catheterization during the night. Nighttime catheterization, if required, should be coordinated with the turning schedule for skin protection. Clinicians should discuss these issues with patients and prospective caregivers.

Persons with SCI who perform self-catheterization may utilize a clean technique. Sterile catheterization is not required. The terminal end of the urethra is colonized by normal flora

Table 2
Medications That Reduce Urethral Outflow Resistance

Medication	Brand Name	Initial Dose	Maximum Dose	Mechanism	Precautions
terazosin	Hytrin	1mg qhs	5 mg bid	alpha-1 antagonist	hypotension sedation headaches syncope
doxazosin	Cardura	1mg qd	16 mg qd	alpha-1 antagonist	hypotension sedation headache syncope
tamsulosin	Flomax	0.4 mg qd	0.8 mg qd	alpha-1A antagonist	no significant hypotension in non-SCI patients retrograde ejaculation nausea diarrhea headache
prazosin	Minipress	1 mg bid	5 mg tid	alpha-1 antagonist	hypotension sedation headache

in all individuals. Even with strict sterile catheterization, these microorganisms will be introduced into the bladder.

Many tetraplegics do not have adequate upper extremity function to independently perform intermittent self-catheterization or other tasks associated with bladder management (i.e., undressing, transfers, disposing of urine, etc.). In some cases, a less than optimal bladder management program is provided because of the lack of human or financial resources. For example, a C5 tetraplegic may benefit from an ICP; however, if a competent caregiver is unavailable to perform the procedure, then other bladder management strategies must be considered.

ICP is not appropriate for patients with urethral pathology, such as false passages and strictures. A successful ICP program requires a bladder capacity of at least 200 cc. In addition, ICP should be avoided in patients who experience autonomic dysreflexia with catheterization.

Indwelling Catheter

A less ideal alternative to an ICP is an indwelling catheter such as a Foley or suprapubic catheter. An indwelling catheter is indicated for an individual who is unable or unwilling to engage in an ICP. Some individuals who have vesicoureteral reflux or significant

incontinence refractory to other treatment strategies may also benefit from an indwelling catheter. Foley catheters are associated with bladder stones, prostatitis and epididymitis, as well as urethral strictures. An indwelling catheter should be changed every two to four weeks. A suprapubic catheter is preferred, as the incidence of epididymitis and prostatitis are decreased. Sexual intercourse is more easily facilitated with a suprapubic catheter when compared with a Foley catheter. As individuals with indwelling catheters (both Foley and suprapubic) have an increased risk of transitional cell and squamous cell carcinoma of the bladder, a cystoscopy every two years is recommended.

Clamping of the Foley

Clamping of the Foley catheter has been advocated as a method of "bladder retraining." This intervention is not recommended, as it may lead to overdistention of the bladder, contribute to urinary tract infections, and may precipitate autonomic dysreflexia.

Pathophysiology of Urinary Tract Infection

Urinary tract infections (UTI) are generally caused by the endogenous flora of the host overcoming other competing normal flora and host defense mechanisms. The presence of the urinary tract infection is affected by the virulence of the invading microorganism, the condition of the urine as the culture medium, and the host defense mechanisms. In healthy individuals, there is a critical balance between the microorganism virulence factors and host defense mechanisms. These virulence factors become less important when the host defense mechanisms are compromised by catheterization or immunosuppression.

Colonization is the growth of microorganisms in the urine without tissue invasion. In contrast, a urinary tract infection is the microbial colonization of urine with associated tissue invasion of the uroepithelium. Persons with SCI are at risk for UTI for a number of reasons. Many individuals are colonized with nosocomial organisms. In addition, elevated post void residual urinary volumes favor bacterial growth. ICP programs introduce bacterial flora from the urethra on a regular basis. A few patients are immunocompromised.

Many common urinary pathogens (i.e., E. Coli or Proteus) possess surface projections known as fimbriae. These projections adhere to the uroepithelium and increase the virulence of the organism. Some bacteria also contain extracellular proteins that resist phagocytosis.

In general, an acidic concentrated urine inhibits microbial growth. Urinary tract infections are prevented by the "wash out" effect of large volumes of urine. The large flow of fluid impedes the adherence of microorganisms and dilutes the concentration of microorganisms. However, large fluid volumes may decrease urine osmolarity, which favors bacterial growth. In addition, excessive fluids may complicate an intermittent catheterization program. Other defenses against UTI include the mucin coat and Tamm-Horsfall proteins produced in the bladder. Furthermore, IgM, IgA and IgG antibodies secreted by the kidneys provide some added protection.

Management of Symptomatic UTI

The diagnostic criterion for urinary tract infection in SCI remains a source of continuing controversy in clinical practice. Typically, a urinary tract infection is diagnosed when there is a significant amount of bacteria and pyuria associated with clinical

abnormalities typically attributable to a spinal cord injury. These symptoms include fever, frequency and dysuria, as well as foul-smelling urine, unexpected incontinence, and increased spasticity. When UTI is diagnosed on the basis of the clinical presentation and urinalysis abnormalities, antibiotic treatment can be instituted after sending a sample to the laboratory for a culture and sensitivity. A five- to seven-day course of oral treatment is sufficient for uncomplicated lower tract infections. Symptomatic reinfections may require a longer course of treatment. If the UTI is complicated by sepsis, intravenous antibiotics are required. A Foley catheter may be temporarily instituted if fluid intake is excessive and results in unacceptable intermittent catheterization volumes.

Asymptomatic Bacteriuria

Maintaining sterile urine at all times in the SCI population is not feasible. Treating asymptomatic UTI may result in colonization with even more virulent drug resistant organisms. In general, asymptomatic UTI in individuals with indwelling catheters should not be treated. If an ICP is utilized, an asymptomatic bacteriuria with fewer than 50 white blood cells per high-power field should not be treated unless there is evidence of vesicoureteral reflux, hydronephrosis, or growth of urea splitting organisms.

Prophylactic Treatment

The role of prophylactic antibiotics has not been established. Methenamine salts, vitamin C supplementation, and cranberry juice can acidify the urine. However, these interventions have not been demonstrated to be effective prophylactic agents in controlled studies.

Lifetime Urological Care

All patients with SCI should have periodic evaluation of the urological system. This should include a thorough clinical assessment, as well as investigations such as renal ultrasound and urodynamic testing.

Chapter 8

Bowel Management

Susan Biener Bergman

Introduction

Bowel dysfunction in SCI is a major source of morbidity. People with SCI require a carefully planned bowel program that allows for socially acceptable continence and prevents fecal impaction. This chapter reviews the pathophysiologic basis of normal and SCI-related bowel dysfunction. Treatment strategies will also be discussed.

Anatomy and Physiology of the Gastrointestinal Tract

The main function of the gastrointestinal tract (Figure 8.1) is to provide the body with water, nutrients and electrolytes. Food is ingested and mechanically and chemically processed in the mouth. It is digested in the stomach and further processed in the small intestine. Digestive end products are then absorbed in the small intestine and the proximal half of the colon. The colon functions as both a storage area and a processing center for waste products as food moves through the GI tract. It is responsible for the absorption of water, electrolytes and short chain fatty acids from the stool. It also supports the growth of beneficial bacteria, secretes mucus to lubricate the stool, and pushes stool out of the body through the rectum and anus.

The colon is essentially a closed tube that is bound proximally by the ileocecal valve and distally by the anal sphincter. It is composed of smooth muscle oriented in an inner circular and an outer longitudinal layer. In between these layers lay Auerbach's plexus and Meissner's plexus, which provide part of the colon's intrinsic innervation. At the end of the colon, at the rectum, the smooth muscle layers thicken to form the internal anal sphincter (IAS). The external anal sphincter (EAS) consists of a circular band of striated muscle that is part of the pelvic floor. The colon and pelvic floor muscles receive parasympathetic, sympathetic and somatic nerve supply.

The parasympathetic supply to the gastrointestinal tract consists of both cranial (vagus nerve) and sacral (pelvic nerve) divisions. In general, increased parasympathetic tone stimulates the gut wall. Sympathetic innervation of the gut projects through the hypogastric nerve via the superior mesenteric, inferior mesenteric, and celiac ganglia. Sympathetic stimulation relaxes the gut wall, ileocecal valve and the IAS. Somatic nerve supply comes from the pudendal nerve (S2 to S4), which supplies the EAS and the pelvic floor musculature.

Intrinsic innervation of the gut is provided by the myenteric plexus (Auerbach's plexus), which lies between the muscle layers and serves primarily a motor function, and the submucosal plexus (Meissner's plexus), which serves primarily a sensory function. Stimulating the myenteric plexus increases the activity of the gut, including increased force and velocity of contractions. The submucosal plexus plays an important role in

coordinating gut wall movements, as well as the secretion of digestive juices.

Two types of movements occur in the digestive tract and are equally important: mixing movements, which agitate intestinal contents and facilitate extraction of nutrients, and peristaltic movements to propel the food bolus toward the rectum and out of the body when the extraction process is complete. Coordination of these movements takes place by three mechanisms: chemical control via neurotransmitters and hormones (i.e., substance P, gastrin and cholecystokinin), neurogenic control via the enteric reflexes (i.e., gastrocolic and rectocolic reflexes), and myenteric control. Since individual smooth muscle fibers in the gut lie very close to one another and some of the membranes are actually fused, the fibers can function as a syncytium through which electrical signals are easily propagated from one fiber to the next. Colonic movements can either involve large sections of the gut (peristalsis), or they can be relatively localized (mixing movements).

Defecation in the Neurologically Intact Individual

The defecation process normally starts when stool is pushed into the rectum by peristalsis. The volume of stool stretches the puborectalis muscle as well as the rectal wall, stimulating the urge to defecate. Voluntary relaxation of the external anal sphincter and the puborectalis muscle straighten the anorectum, allowing for the passage of stool. Stool is pushed out with a combination of continued peristalsis and increased intra-abdominal pressure via the Valsalva maneuver.

Defecation in the Spinal Cord Injured Individual

The SCI individual typically loses both the sensation of rectal fullness and the ability to voluntarily relax the EAS. Depending on the level and completeness of the injury, one of two patterns of bowel dysfunction is seen. In lesions above the conus medullaris, an upper motor neuron (hyperreflexic) bowel is present. The EAS cannot be voluntarily relaxed and the pelvic floor muscles become spastic. However, nerve connections between the spinal cord and colon, as well as the myenteric plexus, remain intact and the stool can be propelled by reflex activity. In lesions below the conus medullaris, a lower motor neuron (areflexic) bowel is present. The myenteric plexus coordinates the movement of stool, but it tends to be quite slow. Most SCI patients experience constipation and, on occasion, fecal impaction. Fecal incontinence is relatively infrequent.

Management of Neurogenic Bowel Dysfunction in Spinal Cord Injury

Although the goals of a treatment plan must be individualized for each patient, the following is a general discussion of a reasonable bowel care program. Prior to instituting a bowel program, premorbid and current bowel function must be ascertained. Pre-existing conditions, including laxative dependency, autonomic neuropathy (i.e., secondary to diabetes), irritable bowel syndrome, or inflammatory bowel disease, may alter gut transit time. These diseases may also diminish the effectiveness of bowel care medications.

For most people with SCI, a complete bowel evacuation every other day is satisfactory. Less frequent bowel movements may result in fecal impaction. For most tetraplegics, a caregiver is needed to complete the bowel regimen. Furthermore, a bowel evacuation may take up to two hours to complete. As such, the bowel program must be scheduled at a time convenient to both patient and caregiver.

When initiating a bowel program, it is worthwhile to begin with an empty colon.

Figure 8.1 **Innervation of the Gastrointestinal System**

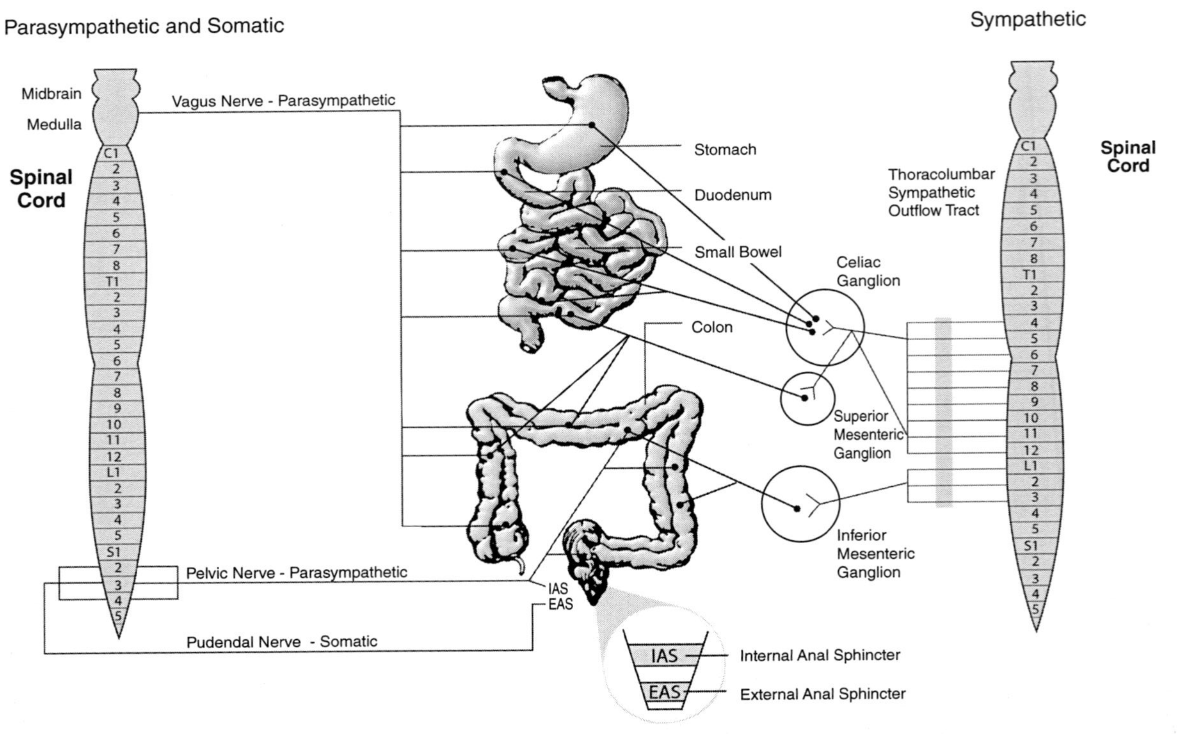

A plain X-ray of the abdomen can be helpful. If obstipation is present, an enema should precede the beginning of the bowel program.

Medications that decrease bowel motility, such as tricyclic agents or narcotics, should be minimized. Broad spectrum antibiotics may inadvertently alter native flora and result in diarrhea. In such cases, consumption of yogurt or lactobacillus preparations (i.e., Lactinex) restore normal gut flora.

Diet

Proper diet is an integral part of successful overall bowel management. Soft bulky stools are more likely to decrease bowel transit time. Toward this goal, the diet should contain adequate amounts of fluids and fiber. Caffeinated beverages, prune juice and apricot nectar can also aid in bowel evacuation. Fatty foods and dairy products, in general, will decrease bowel transit time.

"Fiber" refers to a variety of poorly digestible components of plant material, primarily carbohydrates. There are different types of fiber, which have differing effects on the gastrointestinal tract. These effects are related to the water solubility of the specific type of fiber. In the stomach, dietary fiber tends to prolong gastric emptying time. In the small intestine, fiber can delay absorption of nutrients as well as promote or inhibit stool transit. In the colon, fiber tends to shorten transit time. It provides bulk to stool and eases the transit along the lower bowel, increasing the frequency of bowel movements. This effect is more pronounced with coarsely ground (insoluble) fiber contained in whole grain breads and cereals. Good sources of fiber include whole grain breads and bran cereals. Wheat germ can be added to foods to boost fiber intake if bran cereals are not palatable to the patient. Fruits and vegetables can also provide fiber as well as fluid. An added benefit of a high fiber diet is a feeling of satiety, which may limit the intake of high fat foods.

A careful diet history must be taken to determine the baseline amount of fiber intake. A total of 25 to 35 grams of dietary fiber a day from a variety of sources is probably ideal. This target amount should be achieved gradually. Patients must be closely monitored for any symptoms of intolerance such as unacceptable flatulence, significantly increased stool volume, and painful abdominal distention.

Fluid Intake

Adequate fluid intake (2,500 cc to 3,000 cc per day is ideal) is also essential to a good bowel program. The recommended fluid intake, however, must also be consistent with the bladder management program. Fluid intake should be increased in hot weather or during a febrile illness.

Adjunctive Medications

There are five main classes of medications used to modify bowel habits: stool softeners, colonic stimulants, colonic (contact) irritants, bulk formers, and prokinetic agents (Table 1). The introduction of medications should be individualized. However, stool softeners prevent the formation of hard stools and should be the first-line medication. This should make bowel evacuation easier.

Glycerin and bisacodyl (Dulcolax) suppositories can be useful adjunctive agents in a bowel regimen. Suppositories containing CO2 (such as Magic Bullet) may facilitate

complete emptying in difficult cases. Enemas (e.g., Fleet, Soap Suds) should not be part of a regular bowel program; however, these agents are useful in providing a clear gut prior to beginning a bowel program or for treating fecal obstipation.

Table 1
Sample Oral Adjunctive Bowel Medications

Medication	Brand	Mechanism of Action	Strength	Dose
docusate sodium	Colace	stool softener	100 mg caps	i-ii bid
senna	Senokot	colonic stimulant	8.6 mg tabs	ii qd
bisacodyl	Dulcolax	colonic irritant	5 mg tabs	ii qd
psyllium powder	Metamucil	bulk forming agent	3.4 mg per tsp	i tsp qd-tid
metoclopramide	Reglan	prokinetic agent	10 mg tabs	i qid

Gastrocolic and Rectocolic Reflex

Intact gastrocolic and rectocolic reflexes can be helpful in managing bowel and upper motor neuron bowel dysfunction. The gastrocolic reflex is a normal phenomenon that results in defecation after eating a meal. As such, SCI patients should be placed on the commode within one hour subsequent to a meal. The rectocolic reflex can be manipulated by digital stimulation of the rectum. Digital stimulation is accomplished by gently inserting a lubricated finger into the rectum, and slowly moving the digit in a clockwise manner. A suppository may also be helpful.

Equipment and Positioning

The best position for elimination is sitting upright with the hips and knees flexed on a commode. If possible, the feet should be slightly elevated to place the knees slightly higher than the hips. A less optimal position is the left lateral position in bed. These positions allow for gravity to assist in the flow of stool and place the abdominal muscles at maximum mechanical advantage. A shower commode or patient lift may be required. Care must be taken to prevent pressure ulcers, regardless of whether the bowel evacuation is completed in the bed or on a commode.

Basic Bowel Care Plan for New SCI Patient

- Complete history and physical examination
- Determine goals of bowel program (frequency, timing, location)
- Minimize medications that may decrease bowel motility
- Recommend diet high in fiber, fruits and vegetables
- Minimize fatty foods and dairy products, which may impair gastrointestinal motility
- Standard X-rays of the abdomen to ensure unobstructed bowel
- Introduce stool softener
- Place patient on commode after breakfast to manipulate gastrocolic reflex

- Encourage defecation in sitting position, not in bed
- If no bowel movement, then perform rectal stimulation. If this is unsuccessful, consider suppository
- If no bowel movement after third day, give enema and consider adding second adjunctive medication

Fecal Impaction

The goal of a good bowel regimen is to prevent fecal impaction, which is characterized by absent or diminished passage of stool. Sometimes, overflow diarrhea can be present. Impaction can trigger autonomic dysreflexia, or even lead to a perforated viscus. If impacted stool is present in the rectum, manual disimpaction should be attempted. Anesthetic jelly should be used to prevent autonomic dysreflexia. If the impaction is more proximal, enemas or potent oral stimulants (e.g., magnesium citrate) may be indicated. Surgical consultation may also be indicated. In cases of repeated fecal impaction associated with multiple episodes of dysreflexia, ileostomy or colostomy may be indicated.

Hemorrhoids

Hemorrhoids are usually caused by increased rectal pressure and are often associated with prolonged efforts to remove hard stools. Suppositories, enemas or digital stimulation may exacerbate hemorrhoids. Symptoms include bleeding, pain and autonomic dysreflexia. Effective treatment strategies include maintaining soft stools and regular bowel movements. Topical steroid ointments and medicated suppositories are effective in treating symptoms. If hemorrhoids do not respond to these interventions, then surgical consultation is warranted.

Neurogenic Bowel across the Lifespan

As in the general population, remaining active and maintaining an optimal level of fitness may also help achieve regular and predictable bowel emptying. Aside from lifestyle issues, establishing and maintaining a regular bowel regime will reduce the risk of chronic GI problems, including fecal impaction, hemorrhoids, gastroesophageal reflux disorder, and diverticulosis.

People with SCI are living longer and suffering from many of the diseases that afflict the neurologically intact community, including duodenal ulcers and diverticulitis. They may also develop upper and lower gastrointestinal tract malignancies. Physicians should screen all patients over age 50, including those with SCI, for colorectal cancers with fecal occult blood tests and colonoscopy.

Chapter 9

Pressure Ulcers

Mary Glover

Overview

The SCI population is at significant risk for pressure ulcers. It is estimated that up to 80 percent of SCI individuals will experience a pressure ulcer during their lifetime, and 30 percent will experience recurrent pressure ulcers. A pressure ulcer can profoundly decrease functional independence. In addition, the financial burden to the health-care system can be extraordinary. The vigilance of clinicians is necessary to prevent pressure ulcers. Once an ulcer has formed, rational management strategies may hasten healing and decrease the incidence of complications.

Causation

Pressure ulcers are caused by both extrinsic and intrinsic factors. Extrinsic factors are the external conditions that contribute to ulcer formation, including excessive pressure, shearing, friction and maceration. Intrinsic factors are the conditions that are specific to the individual and include poor nutrition, spasticity, contractures, heterotopic ossification, recurrent urinary tract infection, urinary or fecal incontinence, impaired level of consciousness, substance abuse, and medication intake.

Pressure ulcers are most likely to occur over bony prominences. Common sites include the occiput, scapula, sacrum, ischial bursae, greater trochanter and heel. When tissue pressure exceeds capillary closing pressure, the result is progressive tissue ischemia with concomitant cellular death. The amount of tissue injury is related to the length of time and the amount of pressure the skin experiences.

Shearing forces between the skin and bone cause blood vessels to become angulated and stretched. Consequently, blood flow is compromised, which may result in tissue injury. Friction injury is similar to shearing, in that skin is abraded against the underlying bone and subcutaneous structures. In this case, however, cellular damage is the result of thermal injury. The last significant extrinsic factor is maceration, the softening of the skin secondary to moisture. Urinary incontinence, fecal soiling, and excessive perspiration can lead to maceration.

Prevention

Minimizing extrinsic factors (i.e., pressure, shear, maceration and friction) will decrease the incidence of pressure ulcers. If the patient is confined to bed, the entire skin surface must be assessed daily. To decrease pressure forces, the patient should be turned and positioned every two hours. Padding bony prominences may also be of value (e.g., "sheepskin boots" over heels or a pillow between legs when side-lying). During wheelchair sitting, patients, if capable, should engage in pressure relief strategies (e.g., wheelchair push up, shifting side

to side, tilting or reclining of seating surface, etc.). Proper wheelchair fitting is critical to minimize pressure over seating areas (e.g., ischial bursae).

Shear and friction can be minimized by careful, skilled transfers. When a caregiver moves a patient in bed, care must be taken to avoid excessive shear forces. In SCI, spasticity may exacerbate shear forces and should be managed appropriately. Incontinence of feces and urine can be minimized by physical and pharmacological interventions.

Dressings for Pressure Ulcer Treatment

Table 1

TYPE	**BRAND NAME**
Transparent Films	OpSite Tegaderm Bioclusive
Foams	Allevyn Biatain Lyofoam Mepilex Tielle
Hydrocolloids	DuoDERM Granuflex Comfeel Tegasorb
Alginates	Sorbsan Kaltostat SeaSorb
Antimicrobials	Silvadene Silvarex Aquacel Ag Acticoat Contreet Iodoflex Iodosorb Gel Inadine
Debriding Agents	Santyl (collagenase) ointment
Wound Gels	Intrasite NU-Gel Purilon Gel GranuGEL
Negative Pressure Wound Therapy	EZCARE Engenex Advanced Contratec InfoVAC Invia Liberty/Vario

INDICATION
Generally composed of a polyurethane material and used for partial-thickness wounds, donor sites, and stage I and II pressure ulcers. They are gas permeable and allow moisture vapor to be released, but are not appropriate for wounds with large amounts of exudate. Can be used over bony prominences to reduce friction or sheering.
Generally comfortable, non-adherent to the wound bed, and highly absorbent, allowing for less frequent dressing changes. For use on pressure ulcers, minor burns, skin grafts, diabetic and venous stasis ulcers. Some are available with adhesive borders.
Encourage autologous debridement, insulate the wound bed, and are waterproof, absorbent and impermeable to bacteria, urine and stool. For use on pressure ulcers, venous ulcers and burns. Wound infection is a contraindication.
Highly absorbent, non-adherent and encourage autolytic debridement. Best used on pressure/venous ulcers, wounds with heavy exudates and tunneling. Avoid use on a dry wound bed. Require a secondary dressing.
Antiseptic agent incorporated. Help to reduce risk of infection in partial- and full-thickness wounds. Ability to handle exudate depends on characteristics and composition of product. Metronidazole gel for odor control and anaerobic bacterial control.
For use in acute and chronic wounds requiring debridement, pressure/diabetic ulcers, burns, postoperative wounds, and traumatic or infected wounds.
Provide a moist wound bed healing environment and can help to soften necrotic tissue and promote autolytic debridement. Require a secondary dressing.
FDA class II devices that consist of a vacuum pump, drainage tubing and wound dressing set. For the application of suction (negative pressure) to promote wound healing and for removal of fluids such as wound exudate, irrigation fluids, bodily fluids, or infectious materials. May be indicated for use on chronic, acute, traumatic, subacute and dehisced wounds; diabetic ulcers, pressure ulcers, skin flaps or grafts.

Assessment

Proper documentation of clinical findings enables accurate assessment of improvement or worsening of a lesion. On occasion, a CT scan or MRI may assist in evaluating the depth and severity of a pressure ulcer. Healing or progression of the ulcer should be documented through objective assessment. Objective data include diameter of the ulcer, depth of the ulcer, tissue color, odor, and drainage color.

Figure 9.1 – Staging of Pressure Ulcers

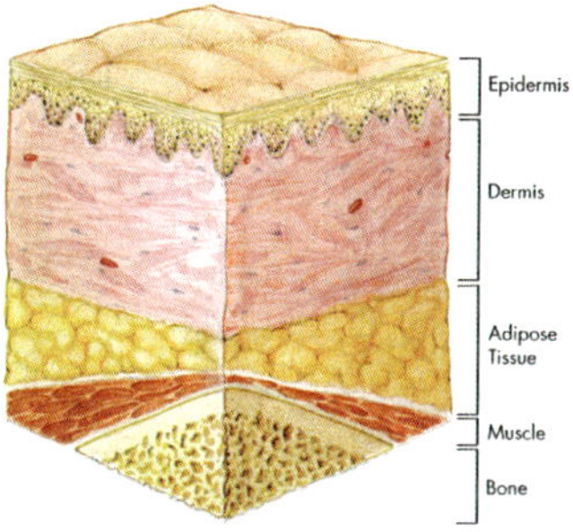

Unstageable – full-thickness tissue loss in which actual depth of the ulcer is completely obscured by slough (yellow, tan, gray, green or brown) and/or eschar (tan, brown or black) in the wound bed; until enough slough and/or eschar are removed to expose the base of the wound, the true depth cannot be determined.

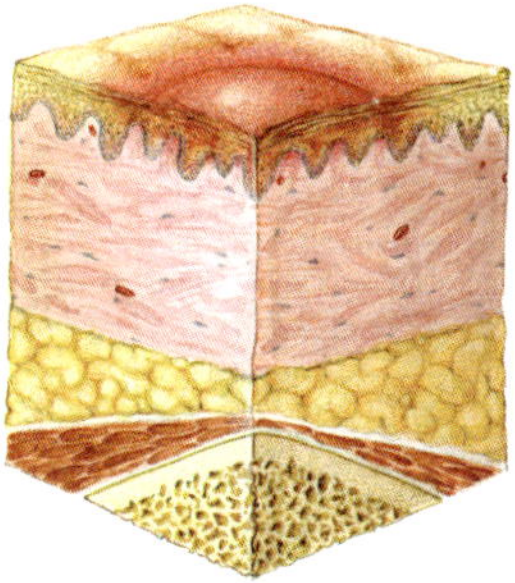

Stage I – intact skin with non-blanchable erythema of a localized area usually over a bony prominence; discoloration of the skin, warmth, edema, hardness or pain may also be present; area may be painful, firm, soft, warmer or cooler compared to adjacent tissue; may be difficult to detect in individuals with dark skin tone.

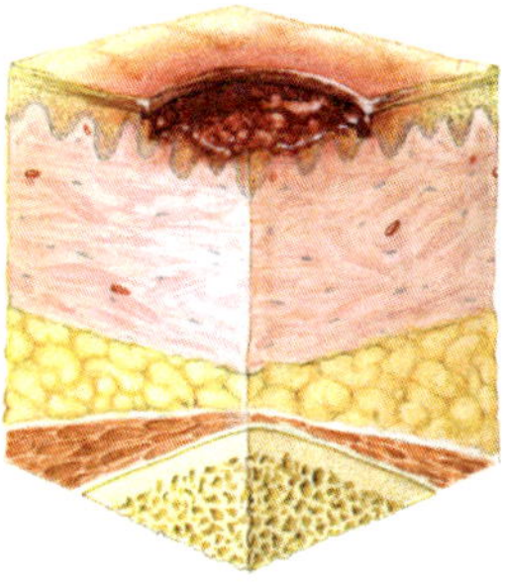

Stage II – partial-thickness loss of dermis presenting as shallow open ulcer with red/pink wound bed, without slough; may also be present as an intact or open/ruptured serum-filled or serosanginous-filled blister; presents as a shiny or dry shallow ulcer without slough or bruising.

Reproduced with permission:

National Pressure Ulcer Advisory Panel and European Pressure Ulcer Advisory Panel. Pressure Ulcer Prevention and Treatment: Clinical Practice Guideline. Washington, DC: National Pressure Ulcer Advisory Panel, 2009.

European Pressure Ulcer Advisory Panel and National Pressure Ulcer Advisory Panel. Pressure Ulcer Prevention and Treatment of: Quick Reference Guide. Washington, DC: National Pressure Ulcer Advisory Panel, 2009.

Stage III – full-thickness tissue loss; subcutaneous fat may be visible but bone, tendon and muscle are not exposed; some slough may be present; may include brimming and tunneling; depth of ulcer varies by anatomical location.

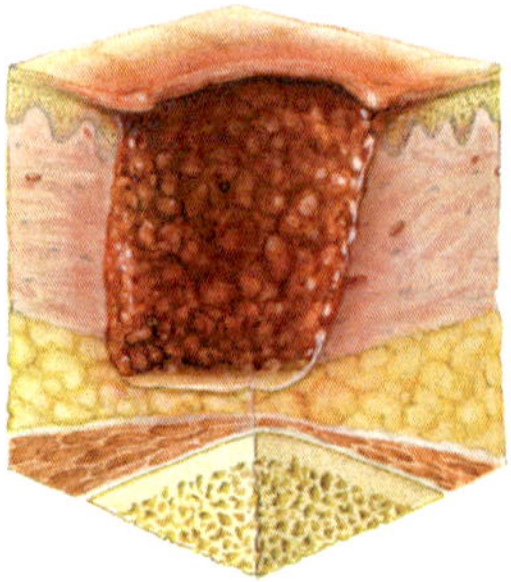

Stage IV – full-thickness tissue loss with exposed bone, tendon or muscle; slough or eschar may be present; often include undermining and tunneling; depth varies by anatomical location; exposed bone/muscle is visible or directly palpable.

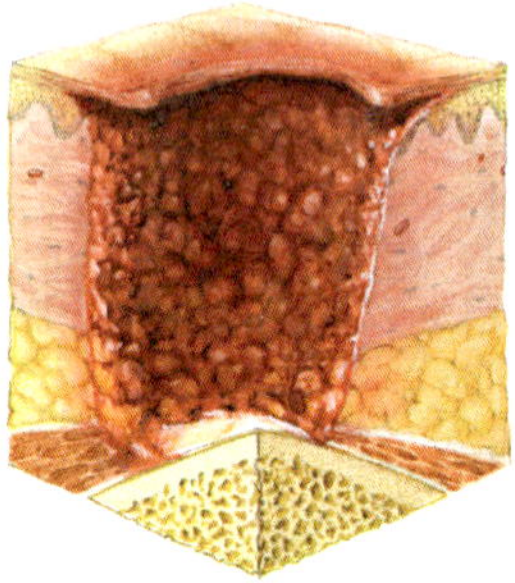

Suspected Deep Tissue Injury – purple or maroon localized area of discolored intact skin or blood-filled blister due to damage of underlying soft tissue from pressure and/or shear; area may be preceded by tissue that is painful, firm, mushy, boggy, warmer or cooler compared to adjacent tissue; evolution may include a thin blister over a dark wound bed that may become covered by thin eschar; may be difficult to detect in individuals with dark skin tones.

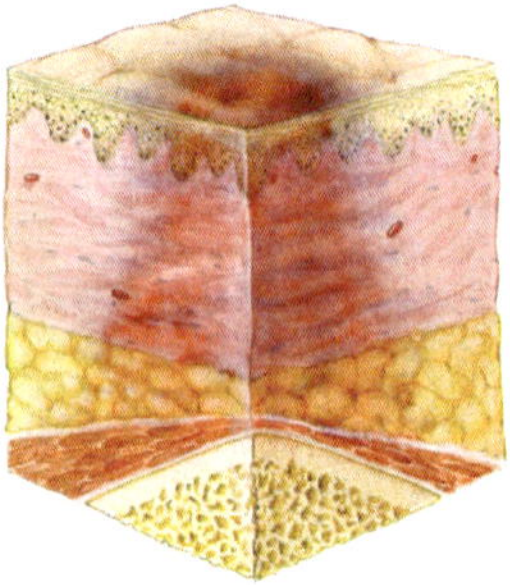

Beds

Proper beds can aid in the prevention and treatment of pressure ulcers. There are several types of bed support surfaces. Static support surfaces, such as foam (Geo-Matt) or static air mattress (Waffle, Sof Care), are an appropriate choice for individuals who have reasonable bed mobility. At a minimum, a static support surface should have one inch of cushion between any bony prominence and the bed frame. Dynamic support surfaces (water, gel, alternating pressure pads), such as an overlay mattress, can be used with individuals who have impaired bed mobility and, therefore, are at high risk of pressure ulcers (e.g., a malnourished, unconscious C5 tetraplegic). These support surfaces are also

appropriate for patients who have Stage I or II ulcers. This type of support surface may also be of value to those who unacceptably compress standard static support surfaces. Low-air-loss (Acucair, KinAir, PneuCare) and air-fluidized (Clinitron, FluidAir) beds may be indicated when a patient has already developed a large Stage III or IV pressure ulcer and has failed to improve with a dynamic overlay. These beds are also helpful for patients who have had a recent surgical flap procedure. Alternate support surfaces are potentially expensive and should only be prescribed as a component of a comprehensive pressure ulcer management program.

Treatment

Every reasonable step should be taken to prevent pressure ulcers. Once a lesion has developed, however, rational treatment should be prescribed. To reduce the progression of the ulcer, the extrinsic factors that contributed to the formation of the ulcer should be identified and treated. In general, healing will be promoted if the wound remains clean, moist and debrided. A non-infected wound will also promote healing.

Management strategies for pressure ulcers can be divided into local and systemic therapies. Local therapies, which are delivered at the pressure ulcer site, include mechanical and chemical treatments. Mechanical methods include wound cleansing, debridement and dressing. Chemical interventions include creams and ointments. Systemic treatments include caloric and vitamin supplementation in addition to intravenous antibiotics.

A pressure ulcer should be cleansed on a regular basis. Normal saline is an excellent cleansing agent. Diluted iodine-based solutions (e.g., Provodine) have germicidal effects; theoretically, this agent impairs wound healing and is not recommended.

Debridement of necrotic tissue will promote wound healing and can be achieved by mechanical or chemical means. Debridement can be achieved by the use of a sharp instrument to remove the debris or devitalized tissue. Other mechanical methods include wet-to-dry gauze dressings, whirlpool therapy, wound irrigation, and dextranomers.

Autolytic debridement occurs when a synthetic dressing is used to cover the wound. This facilitates the natural enzymes produced by the skin to self-ingest the devitalized tissue. Collagenase compounds (e.g., Elase) are chemical debriding agents that can be applied to a wound. This method is contraindicated in infected wounds.

The ideal dressing for the pressure ulcer should keep the wound bed moist and the surrounding skin dry (Table 1). The dressing should control exudate and eliminate dead space. There are many commercially available dressings. However, there is little evidence to support the superiority of any particular brand. As such, the choice of dressings is partly determined by the experiences and preferences of the practitioner. The table on pages 66–67 provides some guidelines for selecting dressings.

If an ulcer is not healing and there is a clinical suspicion of wound infection (i.e., foul odor, purulent drainage, extensive marginal erythema), then a trial of topical antibiotics for a period of two weeks may be considered. Topical antibiotics are not indicated if the patient has sepsis or osteomyelitis. The topical agent should treat the putative pathologic organism. Examples of frequently used topical treatments are silver sulfadiazine, triple antibiotic (neomycin, polymyxin B and bacitracin), and metronidazole cream. Wound cultures are of questionable value, as they may reflect colonization and not the putative pathological organism. Topical antibiotics are available in ointments and creams. Ointments are non-water soluble and should be used with caution because they may impair wound

drainage. If a wound appears infected on clinical grounds, and has not responded to topical antibiotics, a trial of systemic antibiotics may be considered.

Hospitalization and intravenous antibiotics are indicated for complications such as sepsis, advancing cellulitis or osteomyelitis. Osteomyelitis is sometimes difficult to diagnose. Bone biopsy is the "gold standard" for diagnosis. Abnormalities may also be recognized on MRI, bone scan and plain X-rays. Furthermore, the erythrocyte sedimentation rate and white blood cell (WBC) counts may be elevated. The proper management of osteomyelitis requires the involvement of plastic surgery, orthopedic surgery, and infectious disease services. Long-term intravenous antibiotics and possible surgical debridement may be required.

The healing of any wound requires adequate calories, proteins and vitamins. Malnourished individuals should receive dietary supplements (e.g., Ensure, Sustacal). Vitamin C, vitamin A and zinc supplementation may assist with wound healing (Table 2). A nutritionist can formulate an acceptable dietary plan. Caloric intake should be based on ideal body weight (IBW), which is calculated by the following formula:

IBW for males = 50 kg + [2.3 x (height in inches - 60)]
IBW for females = 45.5 kg + [2.3 x (height in inches - 60)]

There is some evidence that biophysical modalities may be an effective component of a pressure ulcer treatment plan. Electrical stimulation and pulsed electromagnetic field treatment may be effective in the treatment of stage II, III and IV ulcers. Ultrasound may be an effective treatment for stage III and IV ulcers. Negative pressure therapy (wound vac) may be used for stage III and IV ulcers.

Stage III and IV ulcers may require surgical treatment. A number of surgical procedures are available, including direct closure, skin grafts, skin flaps, and musculocutaneous flaps. The general medical condition of the patient, as well as the extent of the ulcer, will guide the treatment team. Surgical success is enhanced by ensuring adequate nutrition, treating spasticity, smoking cessation, and control of wound and urinary tract infections prior to surgery. Postoperative care requires a supervised "seating protocol" after a minimum of two weeks of bed rest. Tolerance to pressure is promoted by slowly increasing sitting time, while closely assessing the surgical site for erythema that does not resolve within 10 minutes of pressure relief. Patient education programs for pressure ulcer prevention are essential to long-term success.

Strategies To Prevent Pressure Ulcers

- Vigilant daily skin surveillance
- Turn and position every two hours
- Minimize friction, shear and moisture
- Pad bony prominences
- Encourage early safe mobilization
- Optimize nutrition

Treatment of Pressure Ulcers

- Identify and accurately stage ulcers
- Minimize pressure time, shear, moisture, friction
- Consider alternative bed surface
- Optimize caloric and protein intake
- Zinc, vitamin C, vitamin A supplementation
- Cleanse wound regularly
- Gentle debridement
- Treat infection
- Dressings should be moist and fill empty space
- Skin around wound should be dry
- Surgical consultation for Stage III and IV ulcers

Table 2
Nutritional Interventions For Pressure Ulcer Management

Intervention	Rationale	Dose
protein	necessary for collagen synthesis	Stage II 1.0 – 1.2 gm/kg/day of IBW
		Stage III 1.2 – 1.3 gm/kg/day of IBW
		Stage IV 1.4 –2.0 gm/kg/day of IBW
calories	aids in tissue defense and wound repair	Stage II 25 – 30 calories/day of IBW
		Stage III 30 – 35 calories/day of IBW
		Stage IV 35 – 40 calories/day of IBW
zinc oxide	cofactor for collagen synthesis	25 - 50 mg daily
vitamin C	aids in collagen synthesis	500 - 1000 mg daily
vitamin A	for stimulation of epithelial tissue	20,000 - 25,000 IU daily

Chapter 10

Contracture Management

Steven Nussbaum

Pathology

Contractures are defined as a fixed loss of passive joint range of movement secondary to pathology of connective tissue, tendons, ligaments, muscles, joint capsules or cartilage. Traumatic, inflammatory, ischemic or infectious factors can cause collagen proliferation. These collagen fibers may initially be deposited in a disorganized manner. If the joint is taken through full functional range (either actively or passively), the newly-deposited collagen will organize in a linear fashion. Alternatively, if the joint is immobilized, the collagen matrix will organize in a tightly packed manner, and a contracture will result.

Classification

Contractures can be classified as arthrogenic, soft tissue or myogenic. Arthrogenic contractures are caused by pathology involving the intrinsic joint components. Examples include cartilage damage secondary to osteoarthritis, or joint incongruency as the result of an intra-articular fracture. Arthrogenic contractures generally cause range of movement restrictions in multiple directions.

Soft tissue contractures result in the shortening of tendons, ligaments and skin. These contractures generally cause restriction of movement in one direction.

Myogenic contractures can be divided into intrinsic and extrinsic lesions. Intrinsic muscle contractures are secondary to a primary disorder of muscle fibers. An example would be muscular dystrophy in which histologically abnormal muscle is present. Most traumatic SCI patients suffer from extrinsic muscle contractures as the result of muscles being placed in a shortened position for extended periods of time. The muscle, however, is histologically normal. Factors that can lead to extrinsic contractures include spasticity, immobility, improper positioning and pain. Heterotopic ossification can also cause extrinsic myogenic contractures.

Common Locations of Contractures

In the lower extremities, ankle plantar flexion, hip flexion, and knee flexion contractures are common. In the upper extremities, elbow flexion and supination contractures are possible, depending on the level of injury. Some patients also may develop shoulder adduction and internal rotation contractures. Muscles that cross multiple joints, such as the biceps, hamstrings, tensor fascia lata, and gastrocnemius, are predisposed to contracture formation.

Beneficial Contractures

Some contractures may improve functional status and thus should be encouraged

to develop. For example, C6 tetraplegics have intact wrist extension. This allows the utilization of the tenodesis effect in which active movement of one joint results in the passive movement of other joints. In C6 tetraplegia, the active extension of the wrist (due to an intact extensor carpi radialis) causes passive flexion of the MCP, PIP and DIP joints.

Shortening of the paralyzed flexor digitorum profundus and superficialis will facilitate this passive flexion. This results in a type of prehension that will increase functional independence. To achieve this tenodesis effect, the MCP, PIP and DIP joints must be allowed to contract in slight flexion (approximately 20 degrees). A wrist-driven hinge orthosis (e.g., the RIC or TIRR Orthosis), which stabilizes the thumb, index finger and middle finger, will further promote tenodesis. A biceps flexion contracture may also be useful. When an individual has poor biceps strength, a slight elbow flexion contracture may improve the mechanical advantage of the muscle.

Prevention of Disadvantageous Contractures

Contractures can be prevented with early mobilization, range of movement exercises, proper positioning, and orthotic devices. Contracture prevention requires the coordinated effort of the medical, nursing and therapy services. Patients must be encouraged to get out of bed as soon as practical. The therapeutic exercise program must be tailored to the patient's level of injury. If the patient is capable, ambulation with devices should be encouraged. Patient and caregiver education emphasizing the importance of performing a home stretching program is essential.

Splinting is an effective adjunctive treatment for contracture management. It is not, however, a substitute for a comprehensive rehabilitation treatment program. Orthotic devices can be prescribed to maintain positioning of the hands, elbows, knees and ankles. Patient comfort is essential for a successful splinting program. Skin irritation and pain can result in non-compliance. After initial fabrication of the orthosis, the patient should be monitored every 30 minutes for problems with skin tolerance. If pressure areas are not detected, a two-hour wearing schedule is initiated. The patient may increase the wearing schedule to a full night as skin tolerance allows.

Improper bed positioning may contribute to contractures. The supine position promotes the formation of hip flexion and ankle plantarflexion contractures. Placing a pillow under a patient's knees will promote hip and knee flexion contractures. Another bed position to avoid is one that encourages extreme adduction and internal rotation of the shoulder. Proper bed positioning can minimize contracture formation. Patients should be advised to lie prone in bed to minimize hip flexion contractures. When in bed, the shoulder should be placed in abduction and some external rotation. This can be achieved with strategic placement of pillows. The progression of ankle flexion contractures can be prevented with ankle foot orthosis. Flexion and supination contractures at the elbow can be prevented with resting night splints or bivalved casts, both of which promote elbow extension and pronation.

Proper wheelchair seating and positioning is also essential in preventing the formation of contractures. Contractures and subluxation of the shoulder can be prevented with the placement of armrests and lapboards on the wheelchair. Forward placement of the armrest encourages extension of the elbow.

The pelvis should be maintained with a slight anterior tilt, thus encouraging normal lordosis in the lumbar spine and kyphosis in the thoracic spine. A posterior pelvic tilt

will encourage kyphosis of the lumbar spine, causing the head and neck to lean forward. Extensions, also called hip blocks, placed on a wheelchair laterally keep the pelvis symmetrical and help to align the lower extremities. A short hip block stabilizes the pelvis while a long hip block prevents excessive abduction. Leg straps can be used to prevent adduction of the lower extremities while sitting in the wheelchair. Footrest height can be adjusted to change the position of the ankle, knee and hip. The trunk can be stabilized by utilizing laterally placed trunk supports and by modifying the seat to recline 10 degrees.

Treatment of Contractures

Every reasonable step should be taken to prevent contractures. Once a contracture has formed, however, a variety of interventions are available. The factors that are contributing to contracture formation, such as pain, spasticity, inflammation and improper positioning, should be treated. Treatments can be divided into three groups: physical, medical and surgical.

Physical interventions include therapeutic heat (i.e., ultrasound) prior to a stretching program. A terminal sustained stretch is essential. Caution must be used with therapeutic heat in areas with impaired sensation. Regional osteoporosis may also have caused fragile bones, and vigorous stretching may lead to a fracture.

Figure 10.1 **Serial Casting**

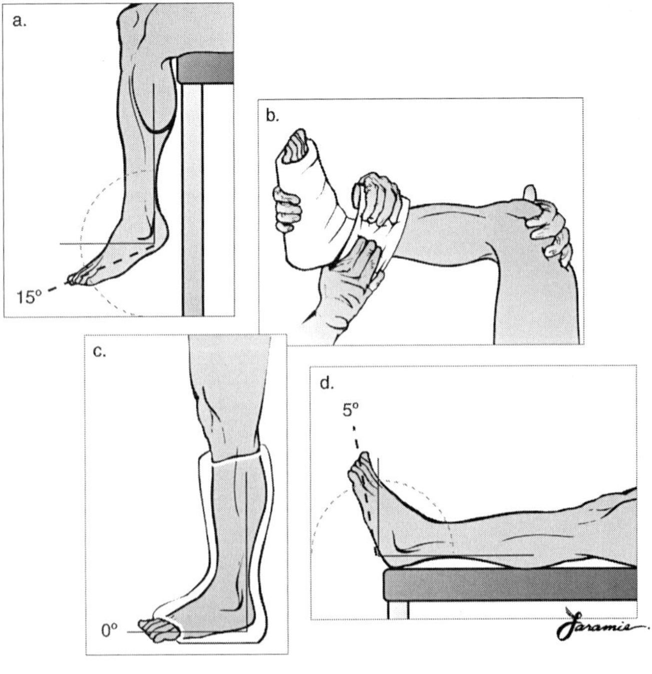

Serial casting or dynamic splinting can be an adjunctive therapy to a stretching program. Serial casting (Figure 10.1) utilizes a plaster cast that is applied to a limb that has been pre-stretched approximately five degrees. The cast is subsequently removed in three to five days, and a new cast is placed after the limb is stretched another five to 10 degrees. This process continues until the contracture has been reduced. Serial casting should be discontinued if pain or pressure ulcers develop. Dynamic splinting utilizes splints with movable parts to counter contracting forces. Dynasplints and outrigger splints are examples of dynamic splints.

In refractory cases, orthopedic surgical procedures, such as joint manipulation, tendon release, and tendon lengthening, can be considered. If pain or spasticity are contributing to contractures, these conditions should be managed appropriately. These topics are discussed in other chapters of this monograph.

Chapter 11

Autonomic Dysfunction

Nancy DeSantis

SCI compromises the motor, sensory and autonomic pathways. Impairment of the motor tracts leads to weakness, whereas impairment of the sensory tracts leads to dysesthesias and anesthesia. Dysfunction of the autonomic pathways is associated with the clinical findings of autonomic dysreflexia such as severe hypertension and headaches. Other dysautonomic features include baseline hypotension, orthostatic hypotension, impaired thermoregulation, and diminished sweating.

Cardiovascular Function

Blood pressure is the product of cardiac output and total peripheral resistance. Cardiac output is the product of heart rate and stroke volume. Stroke volume is directly related to cardiac venous return. Heart rate and blood pressure are influenced by the effects of the sympathetic and parasympathetic nervous system. In SCI, the parasympathetic vagus fibers, which originate in the brain stem, are usually spared. However, the sympathetic fibers, which originate in the thoracic and lumbar spinal cord, may be disrupted by SCI, depending on the level of injury.

Table 1
Medications to Treat Hypotension in SCI

Generic Name	Brand Name	Initial Dose	Maximum Dose	Mechanism	Precautions
fludrocortisone acetate	Florinef	0.1 mg	0.4 mg	mineralocorticoid that promotes sodium and water retention	hypertension, CHF, hypokalemic alkalosis, peripheral edema, hypernatremia
ephedrine sulfate	Ephedrine	25 mg bid	50 mg tid	alpha and beta agonist	tachycardia, arrhythmias, palpitations, headache, urinary retention, insomnia, sweating, tremulousness
midodrine hcl	ProAmatine	2.5 mg tid	10 mg tid	alpha-1 agonist	headache paresthesias dysuria pruritus piloerection

Hypotension

Hypotension can present in the acute and/or chronic phase of SCI. Hypotension is related to decreased vascular tone, diminished circulating catecholamines, and impaired venous return. An orthostatic component is frequently identified. It is not unusual for patients to have sitting systolic blood pressures in the 60 mm Hg - 80 mm Hg range. Some individuals experience dizziness and syncope, whereas others are asymptomatic. Symptoms may be exacerbated by meals, as blood is shunted to the gastrointestinal system for digestion. Symptoms may be exacerbated with exercise. Treatments include thigh high compression stockings and abdominal binders. Caregivers should slowly sit persons with SCI from the recumbent position. If these strategies are unsuccessful, fludrocortisone, ephedrine and midodrine can be considered.

Table 2

Medications to Treat Chronic Dysreflexia

Medication	Brand Name	Initial Dose	Maximum Dose	Mechanism	Precautions
phenoxybenzamine	Dibenzyline	10 mg bid	40 mg tid	alpha antagonist	avoid alcohol postural hypotension tachycardia nasal congestion miosis
clonidine (oral) or clonidine (weekly patch)	Catapres Catapres TTS	0.1 mg qd 0.1 mg/24 h	0.8 mg tid 0.3 mg/24 h	central acting alpha-2 agonist	orthostatic hypotension withdrawal hypertension sedation constipation dry mouth weakness skin rash pruritus tricyclics may decrease effectiveness
terazosin	Hytrin	1mg qhs	10 mg bid	alpha-1 antagonist	hypotension sedation headaches fatigue syncope
prazosin	Minipress	1 mg bid	5 mg tid	alpha-1 antagonist	hypotension sedation headache fatigue syncope

Impaired Thermoregulation

Maintenance of normal body temperature requires an intact autonomic and neuroendocrine system. Thermoregulation is coordinated by the hypothalamus. When core body temperature is decreased, homeostatic mechanisms cause shivering. In addition, blood flow to the extremities is reduced. When core body temperature is elevated, the normal homeostatic response is to increase sweating and to shunt blood toward the extremities. In SCI, these normal regulatory mechanisms may be dysfunctional due to compromised autonomic pathways. Hyperthermia and hypothermia are common. Prior to concluding that a patient has hyperthermia (i.e., quad fever) secondary to dysautonomia, other causes of fever should be excluded. High fevers are rarely, if ever, due to quad fever. It is not uncommon that hyperthermia and hypothermia are related to ambient temperature (poikilothermia) and may be corrected by adjusting the thermostat. Individuals with impaired thermoregulation should have homes and vans that have excellent climate control systems.

Autonomic Dysreflexia

Autonomic dysreflexia (AD) is a syndrome characterized by a sudden rise in systolic and diastolic blood pressure in response to noxious stimuli below the level of injury. It is most often associated with bradycardia. However, tachycardia and other cardiac rhythm disturbances are possible. Other symptoms include sweating or flushing above the level of the injury, pallor below the level of injury, sudden pounding bilateral headache, nasal congestion, anxiety, and, rarely, visual disturbances. Typically, AD is associated with injuries at or above the T6 level; however, there are cases reported with lower thoracic lesions. The elevations in blood pressure may range from 20 mm Hg (systolic and/or diastolic) above the baseline to in excess of 200 mm Hg systolic and 100 mm Hg diastolic. Silent AD may not cause symptoms, but should be noted when systolic blood pressure rises 20 mm HG to 40 mm HG above baseline. Untreated AD can lead to intracerebral hemorrhage, seizure or death.

Autonomic dysreflexia occurs after the period of spinal shock has resolved. Individuals must have an intact spinal cord below the level of injury to develop AD. Noxious stimuli below the neurological level travel to the spinal cord and cause reflex sympathetic constriction of the vascular structures. This may result in increased preload and resultant hypertension. The elevated blood pressure is detected by the carotid baroreceptors, which results in increased vagal tone. This usually results in bradycardia. However, heart rate is influenced by the opposing effects of the sympathetic and parasympathetic systems. As such, tachycardia is also possible. In uninjured persons, this

Table 3
Common Causes of Autonomic Dysreflexia

Bladder distention	Bladder stones	Ingrown toenails	Cystoscopy
Fecal impaction	Skin ulcers	Bone fractures	Gastric ulcers
Urinary tract infection	Epididymitis Cholecystitis	Restrictive clothing	Detrusor sphincter dyssynergia
Kidney stones			

reflex vascular constriction is modulated by higher brain stem, subcortical and cortical centers. This modulation, however, is absent or impaired in persons with SCI.

To manage autonomic dysreflexia, the precipitating cause must be identified and treated. The individual should be placed in the sitting position in order to induce venous pooling and decrease preload. Blood pressure should be monitored every five minutes. The patient should be catheterized to alleviate a distended bladder. Constricting garments or devices should be removed. Search for any sharp objects pressing into the skin. Position the patient to alleviate pressure if there is skin breakdown. Pre-treat with Lidocaine jelly, then perform a rectal exam to check for bowel distention or impaction. If the systolic blood pressure is above 150 mm Hg and the precipitant cause cannot be readily treated, medical therapy should be instituted. Topical or sublingual nitrates are appropriate choices.

Topical nitroglycerin has a rapid onset and should be applied above the level of the lesion. If hypotension results, the nitropaste should be wiped away and the individual should be placed in a recumbent position with the legs elevated. If dysreflexia cannot be controlled, admission to an intensive care unit for intravenous nitroglycerin or nitroprusside should be considered. It should be noted that nitrates should not be prescribed if the patient used a phosphodiesterase 5 inhibitor in the previous 24 hours. Examples of these agents include sildenafil (Viagra), vardenafil (Levitra), and tadalafil (Cialis). In such cases, oral nifedipine can be considered. Sublingual nifedipine should not be administered because its use can result in severe hypotension and stroke.

Chronic Autonomic Dysreflexia

Chronic autonomic dysreflexia develops in some individuals. Successful management requires the recognition and treatment of precipitating conditions (i.e., bladder spasticity, pressure ulcers, renal or bladder calculi, etc.). There are a number of medications that may be utilized to manage chronic autonomic dysreflexia (Table 2). However, medications may also lower baseline blood pressure and contribute to orthostatic hypotension.

Chapter 12

Upper Motor Neuron Syndrome and Spasticity

Mark Kaplan

The upper motor neuron syndrome consists of positive and negative findings. Positive manifestations include spasticity, athetosis, primitive reflexes, rigidity and dystonia. Negative findings include weakness, paralysis and fatigue.

Spasticity, an abnormality of muscle tone, becomes clinically apparent as spinal shock resolves. It is characterized by a velocity-dependent resistance to passive joint movement. Other clinical findings include hyperactive muscle stretch reflexes and clonus. Many persons with SCI also experience flexor and cutaneo-motor spasms. Although these abnormalities of motor control are not considered manifestations of spasticity, they may respond to many of the same management strategies. In the chronic phase of SCI, an increase in spasticity or spasms may be secondary to medical complications such as urinary tract infection, bowel impaction or syrinx.

Measuring Spasticity

The Ashworth and Modified Ashworth Scales are the most commonly used scoring instruments and are based on findings during clinical examination. The Spasm Frequency Score is based on the reporting of the individual experiencing abnormalities in muscle tone. Researchers use electrophysiological parameters, such as F-wave and H-reflex measurements (threshold, latency, amplitude, etc.), to quantify spasticity. However, changes in electrophysiological measures may not correlate with clinical or functional improvements. Some studies have utilized the pendulum test, as well. This test involves placing the examinee in a supine position with the legs hanging over the edge of the plinth. The leg is allowed to fall, and knee movement is assessed with an electrogoniometer.

Modified Ashworth Scale

- 0 = No increase in muscle tone
- 1 = Slight increase in muscle tone, manifested as a catch-and-release or by minimal resistance at the end of range of motion
- 1+ = Slight increase in muscle tone, manifested by catch, followed by minimal resistance throughout the remainder (less than half) of the range of motion
- 2 = More marked increase in muscle tone through most of the range of motion, but the affected part is easily moved
- 3 = Considerable increase in muscle tone; passive movement difficult
- 4 = Affected part(s) rigid

Spasm Frequency Score

0 = No spasms
1 = Mild spasm induced by stimulation
2 = Infrequent, full spasm occurring less than once per hour
3 = Spasms occurring more than once per hour
4 = Ten or more spasms per hour, or continuous contraction

Contracture and Spasticity

Many times, contracture and spasticity coexist in SCI. Increased tone leads to diminished movement. The result is a cycle that, if untreated, can have deleterious consequences.

Upper Motor Neuron Syndrome and Function

Not all the manifestations of the upper motor neuron syndrome require treatment. Sometimes, spasticity and spasms can be beneficial. For example, a patient may use knee extensor spasticity to assist in transferring from a sitting to standing position. Spasticity of knee extensors may also increase stability during the stance phase of gait. Spasms may be used to assist with bed mobility. Alternatively, increased muscle tone can be deleterious. For example, spasticity may contribute to a poor seating position, which could contribute to contractures and skin breakdown. Flexor spasms of the lower extremity may cause a person with SCI to strike a limb against the leg rests of a wheelchair.

Indications for Treatment of Spasticity

Decrease pain	Minimize contractures	Improve seating
Improve nursing care	Assist in prevention and healing of pressure ulcers	Improve gait and transfers
Improve hygiene		Improve self-care activities

Areas of Skin Breakdown Associated With Spasticity

Muscle Group	Area of Potential Skin Breakdown
Shoulder adductors	Axilla
Elbow flexors	Antecubital fossa
Finger flexors	Palm
Hip adductors	Perineum
Knee flexors	Sacrum, heels

Pain and Spasticity

Spasticity may produce pain directly or due to the prolonged contraction of a muscle. Contractures and pressure ulcers can cause pain, which may increase nociceptive afferent impulses and lead to further spasticity.

Treating Spasticity

The treatments for spasticity include physical, medical and surgical interventions. The first step in treating spasticity is to recognize and manage stimuli that may be

contributing to increased tone such as urinary tract infections, bladder stones, fecal impaction, heterotopic ossification, or pressure ulcers.

Table 1
Anti-Spasticity Medications

Medication	tizanidine	clonidine	dantrolene sodium	diazepam	baclofen
Brand Name	Zanaflex	Catapres (oral) Catapres TTS (weekly patch)	Dantrium	Valium	Lioresal
Mechanism of Action	alpha-2 agonist (centrally acting)	alpha-2 agonist (centrally acting)	Inhibits Ca2+ release	GABA facilitation	GABA analogue
Starting Dose	2 mg bid	0.1 mg PO bid 0.1 mg/24-hour patch	25 mg qd	2.5 mg bid	2.5 mg bid
Maximum Dose*	36 mg/day	2.4 mg/day 0.3 mg/24-hour patch	400 mg/day	60 mg/day	80 mg/day
Common Side Effects	drowsiness weakness dry mouth mild hypotension	weakness sedation constipation skin rash dry mouth pruritus orthostatic hypotension withdrawal hypertension	weakness sedation dizziness paresthesia nausea diarrhea hepatitis	sedation weakness depression ataxia memory loss dependence	sedation fatigue weakness nausea dizziness paresthesia decreased seizure threshold hallucinations and seizures if withdrawn abruptly

Table adapted from Whyte J, Robinson KM. Pharmacologic management. In: Glenn MB, Hyte J, editors. The practical management of spasticity in children and adults. Malvern, PA: Lea and Febinger; 1990: 222.

Positioning

Tone may be affected by head and body positions. The tonic neck and vestibular reflexes may be useful in modulating spasticity. For example, some persons with SCI have diminished tone in the partially recumbent position. As such, this position is incorporated into wheelchair-sitting strategies. Casting or splinting an extremity may also diminish spasticity.

Modalities

Cryotherapy and electrical stimulation can reduce spasticity for several hours after application. Sustained cold over a muscle group (i.e., 20 minutes) may decrease spasticity. Alternatively, quick cooling or electrical stimulation of an antagonist of a spastic muscle group may result in reciprocal inhibition and thereby decrease muscle tone. Many individuals with SCI, however, are insensate below their neurological level, and modalities must be prescribed with extreme caution.

Stretching

A stretching program can minimize tone. It should be incorporated into the individual's daily routine. When stretching muscles, a terminal sustained stretch is essential for diminishing tone. The benefit of stretching may last throughout the day.

Medications

Side effects of medications may limit their use (Table 1). The most commonly used first-line agent is baclofen. However, some experts believe that tizanidine is a more appropriate choice. The annual cost of therapy (medications, required laboratory tests, repeat physician visits, etc.) should be considered in treatment decisions.

Nerve Blocks

Nerve blocks involve injecting a medication close to a nerve causing temporary or permanent dysfunction (Figure 12.1). A temporary nerve block can be completed with lidocaine or bipivacaine. This may allow a clinician to evaluate the potential benefits of a nerve block and facilitate the use of other interventions such as serial casting or dynamic splinting. To perform a longer acting nerve block (chemical neurolysis) agents such as phenol and ethanol may be employed.

Nerve blocks can be performed at any anatomically accessible nerve. It is possible to block nerve fibers at the root, plexus or peripheral nerve. Some muscle groups (e.g., iliopsoas) cannot be practically blocked at a distal site, so the neurolysis must be completed at the nerve root.

Nerve blocks completed on sensorimotor nerves can result in unwanted dysesthesias and, rarely, anesthesia. However, if the person with SCI is insensate at the site of the nerve block, the potential sensory side effects are less of a concern. Reducing sensory input, however, may be beneficial, as nociceptive inputs sometimes exacerbate spasticity. A motor branch block is a type of chemical neurolysis in which the most distal motor branches of a peripheral nerve are blocked. Motor branch blocks require more needle insertions and can be tedious to perform. There is, however, a lower risk of sensory complications. Other complications from nerve blocks include weakness and sensitivity to the injected agent. Phenol blocks can lead to fibrosis of the nerve and make future nerve blocks at the same site more difficult.

Paravertebral nerve root blocks have more potential side effects. If during a lumbar paravertebral block, the subarachnoid space is inadvertently compromised, incontinence, sexual dysfunction and ascending paralysis are possible.

Figure 12.1 **Potential Nerve Blocks in Lower Extremity**

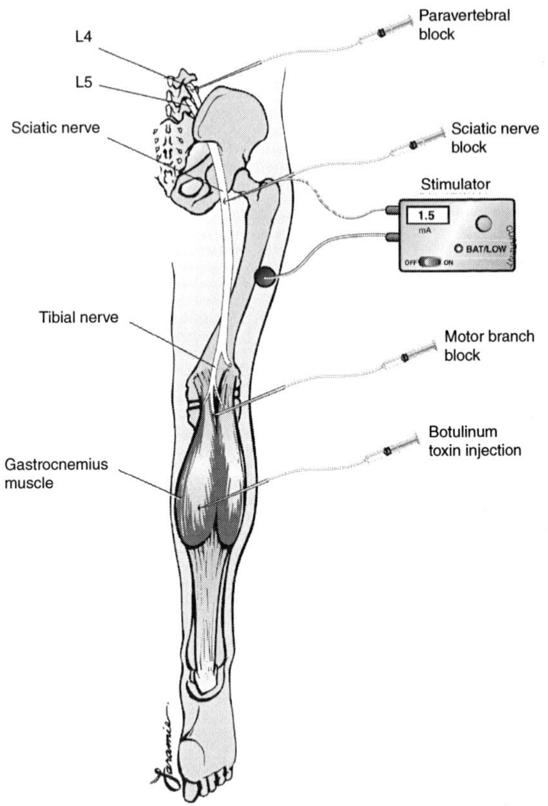

The duration of effect from chemical neurolysis is variable. On average, the effects of the procedure should last between three and nine months. However, in some individuals, the benefits persist for many years. Nerve blocks should be used as part of a comprehensive rehabilitation treatment program; by adding a stretching program, the benefits may be prolonged.

Localization of the nerve is critical for a successful nerve block. The closer the medication is delivered to the nerve, the less medication is required and fewer side effects are likely. The site of injection can be localized with a variable intensity pulse stimulator. A needle coated with Teflon (except at the tip) is attached to a syringe. Current is delivered through the needle by a stimulator. As the needle approaches the nerve, a muscle contraction will be elicited. The closer the needle is to the nerve, the less current will be required. With this technique, the medication can be delivered very close to the nerve.

Nerve blocks are commonly performed on muscles innervated by the median, ulnar, obturator, sciatic and tibial nerves. In general, blocking a motor branch is preferred to a mixed sensorimotor nerve.

Botulinum Toxin

The Clostridium botulinum bacterium produces a neurotoxin. When pharmacological preparations of this agent are injected in muscle fibers, there is inhibition of the release of acetylcholine. The result is a neuromuscular blockade with a subsequent decrease in muscle strength and tone.

There are seven serotypes that are antigenically distinct. Currently, botulinum serotype A and B are commercially available. There are three botulinum A products commercially available: onabotulinumtoxin A (Botox), abobotulinumtoxin A (Dysport), and incobotulinumtoxin A (Xeomin). In the US, the only botulinum toxin B commercially available is rimabotulinumtoxin B (Myobloc).

Botulinum toxin injection, unlike a nerve block, does not require the use of electromyographic localization. However, many clinicians use electromyographic guidance or stimulation to assist in muscle localization. Risks of injection include reaction to the injectant, bleeding and infection. There have been reports of the systemic spread of botulinum toxin, resulting in weakness of muscles distal to the injection, hoarseness of voice, and voiding dysfunction, as well as diplopia, ptosis and dysphagia. This procedure has a duration of effect from one to six months and may be more appropriate for patients soon after injury. The onset of effect typically occurs several days after injection and the maximum effect is obtained over a period of several weeks. This may be of benefit in allowing patients to gradually adapt to their new muscle strength. Disadvantages include the high cost relative to anesthetic or phenol injection.

Baclofen Pump

Intrathecal baclofen delivery may be effective in patients whose spasticity is not controlled by other means. A temporary catheter is placed into the intrathecal space and a 50 microgram test dose of baclofen is given. A 100 microgram dose can be tried if the lower dose is ineffective and there are no significant side effects. If effective, a permanent catheter is implanted. The pump with a reservoir is placed subcutaneously and refilled at one- to three-month intervals. Potential side effects include infection, catheter breakage, drowsiness, hypotension and weakness. With an overdose, respiratory depression is possible. Autonomic dysreflexia can be precipitated if the intrathecal baclofen is abruptly discontinued.

Surgical Treatment

Destructive neurosurgical procedures, such as rhizotomy and cordotomy, are rarely performed. Orthopedic procedures can also be considered in selected cases. Irreversible procedures should not be performed until neurological recovery has plateaued, typically up to one year post-injury.

Chapter 13

Heterotopic Ossification

Douglas E. Garland

The term heterotopic ossification (HO) is preferred to such terms as ectopic ossification, paraosteoarthropathy, or myositis ossificans when discussing the formation of new bone near joints as a consequence of SCI. Heterotopic refers to the occurrence in more than one area. Microscopically, the bone is a true "ossific" process, progressing de novo to new bone formation rather than to calcification of soft tissue.

Genetics and Patient Predisposition

Strong support for some type of genetic predisposition to HO formation is derived from research into the hereditary disorder fibrodysplasia ossificans progressiva (FOP). This disorder is inherited as an autosomal dominant trait with full penetrance and variable expression. It is a disorder of connective tissue, with skeletal malformations and HO. The natural history of HO associated with FOP has similarities to the natural history of HO from other causes, especially neurogenic HO.

The association of human leukocyte antigens (HLA) with neurogenic HO has been documented. An increased prevalence of HLA-B18 and HLA-B27 antigens has been reported in some SCI patients with HO. However, follow-up studies from other centers have not confirmed these findings. This system cannot presently predict susceptibility to HO.

Clinical Presentation

Clinically significant HO (i.e., resulting in significant limitation in joint range) affects approximately 10 percent to 20 percent of SCI patients. Ankylosis occurs in fewer than 10 percent of these lesions. Symptoms of HO are usually recognized within the first two months post-injury. It is unusual for HO to be diagnosed beyond six months post-SCI. HO usually presents in the paralyzed extremities (i.e., below the neurological level).

Clinical findings include erythema, pain and swelling. Other manifestations include decreased joint range of movement, increased spasticity, and low-grade fevers. With incomplete lesions, patients may experience pain. Differential diagnosis includes deep venous thrombosis, cellulitis, abscess, septic joint, hematoma and tumor.

The most common sites for HO in SCI patients are the hips and knees. In the hip, the lesion is usually anterior to the hip joint. It courses in a plane from the anterior iliac spine toward the lesser trochanter. Pseudoarthrosis, which allows for passive movement, is commonly noted. Although HO may occur anywhere in the anterior thigh, it is most commonly noted in the distal anteromedial knee. Ankylosis is uncommon. HO rarely involves the shoulder or elbow. In such cases, the mass is usually small and can be noted in any plane. Other sites are rare.

Diagnosis

Elevated levels of serum alkaline phosphatase (SAP) and creatine phosphokinase (CPK) may be associated with clinically significant HO. This is particularly true at the hip. SAP levels begin to rise to the upper limits of normal within the first two weeks of injury. At three weeks, the SAP levels may exceed normal values, and the elevation may persist for up to five months. The SAP level parallels the clinical course of HO.

The three-phase radionuclide bone scan is the best method for early detection and confirmation of HO. This test requires an intravenous injection of 99mTc-labeled methylene diphosphonate. The radioisotope concentrates in areas of increased bone activity. The three phases of a bone scan are the dynamic blood flow phase (nuclear angiogram), immediate static phase (blood pool phase), and the delayed static phase. Abnormalities in the first two phases of the bone scan will be present prior to abnormalities in the third phase. Clinicians should insist on a three-phase study, and not a single static phase study. A three-phase bone scan can detect HO as early as two to three weeks after the onset of the lesion.

Radiographs may provide confirmatory evidence of HO. Although plain films may detect HO as early as three weeks after injury, radiographic detection may not be confirmatory until two months after the initial clinical presentation.

The precise role of computed tomography (CT) scanning as a clinical tool for diagnosis and a measure of maturation of HO is not established. CT scanning clearly defines HO and its relationship to muscles, vessels and nerves. This study should be considered prior to surgical excision.

Treatment

The clinical significance of HO varies from patient to patient, and management decisions must be individualized. In some individuals, the HO is of little functional significance and requires no intervention. Others suffer from multiple lesions that impair function significantly. The majority of patients can be satisfactorily managed with physical therapy and medications.

Physical Therapy

Physical therapy can be helpful in the management of HO. The goal is to maintain functional range of movement. The affected joints should be gently moved through functional range. Vigorous force, however, should not be used, as this may lead to further ectopic bone formation.

Medical Management

Prophylactic HO treatment with medications for every SCI is probably not warranted. If there is a clinical suspicion of HO, then a bone scan is appropriate.

Patients diagnosed with HO can be treated with etidronate disodium (EHDP). This medication is a structural analog of inorganic phosphate and limits ossification by blocking the formation of hydroxyapatite crystals. The oral dose is 20 mg/kg per day, and may be given in one dose or in two divided doses for a period of up to six months. Some clinicians recommend that initial treatment should be with intravenous EHDP (300 mg per day) for the first three days, followed by oral therapy. The most common side effects of EHDP are nausea, vomiting and diarrhea. In studies with dogs, pathologic fractures

have developed after nine months of treatment.

Nonsteroidal anti-inflammatory drugs (NSAID) have not been studied extensively in HO associated with SCI. They may eventually be proven effective, but presently are adjuncts to EHDP. NSAID may be indicated subsequent to surgical resection. Indomethacin is the preferred NSAID, at 25 mg tid. Alternate choices are ibuprofen 300-400 mg tid and aspirin 650 mg tid.

Surgery

Surgery is appropriate in selected cases that are refractory to conservative management. Surgical indications include functionally impaired joint mobility, impaired sitting, and significant spasticity. Surgical treatment may range from a wedge resection to the complete removal of the lesion. The goal is not to eradicate the ectopic bone, but rather to allow for functional range of movement. Surgery should be planned when the HO is at a quiescent state (i.e., normal SAP levels, mature radiographic appearance, and baseline bone scan). It may take up to 18 months for a lesion to reach this inactive stage. Postoperative prophylaxis is necessary. Combination therapy is desirable. Radiation at 600 - 750 rads in single or divided doses is appropriate. As well, EHDP or NSAID are necessary for a period of three to six months.

Chapter 14

Psychological Adaptation

J. Scott Richards

Psychological Function during Acute Rehabilitation Admission

During the first few weeks to months following SCI, the whole continuum of human emotional responses and defenses against what could be overwhelming reality can be seen. The older rehabilitation literature describes stage theories for this process, which imply a predictable if not necessary sequence of emotional and cognitive reactions as persons with SCI move toward "adjustment." There is, however, no universal path to adjustment. Adjustment is not an end point but a lifelong process of adaptation. However, there are a number of commonly experienced emotional reactions. Often, these reactions become clinically appreciated in the rehabilitation setting, when the individual with SCI initially confronts his limitations.

Depressive behavior is often present. It can be difficult to distinguish between an acceptable reactive depressive episode (i.e., grief secondary to loss of function) as opposed to a problematic major depression. Persistent sadness (dysphoria) in response to the recognition of functional losses is common, appropriate and typically time-limited. Support, encouragement and empathic listening are all helpful responses to this process when it occurs. Deciding when someone has a major depression, however, can be more problematic. Clinical signs of depression, such as sleep disturbance, weight loss, loss of appetite, diminished energy, and diminished interest in sexual functioning, can all be sequelae of medical complications and not directly reflective of a major depressive episode.

Anxiety is often evident as well and, in a smaller proportion of cases, full-blown post-traumatic stress disorder can be seen. Judicious use of anxiolytics can be helpful as a short-term intervention, but needs to be weighed against the implicit message that adjustment to injury can best be done passively through medications rather than actively through coping. If anxiety impairs the learning that is required to participate in the rehabilitation program, then medication should be considered. Behavioral treatment approaches for anxiety should also be considered, including relaxation training and imagery deconditioning techniques.

Other reactions, such as anger, hostility and withdrawal, are often seen as well. However, staff members are often baffled by the lack of apparent negative emotional reactions in some persons with SCI. There is no convincing evidence that the absence of strong negative emotions bodes poorly for the future. Patients need to be assessed carefully to ascertain their true level of psychological distress.

Whether to confront the patient directly with the permanence of his injury is an issue that must be decided without the benefit of empirical data. The clinical consensus seems to be that physicians should directly respond to the patient's questions with regard to

prognosis. If the patient has not requested prognostic information about neurological recovery, it is potentially harmful to the therapeutic relationship to directly confront the individual.

Cognitive Concerns

Given the epidemiology of SCI, with a large percentage of injuries caused by rapid deceleration events (e.g., motor vehicle crashes), there should be a high index of suspicion for concomitant traumatic brain injury. This will be obvious in some cases in terms of impaired memory, judgment, impulse control and reasoning, but may be much more subtle and more difficult to detect in others. Concomitant significant traumatic brain injury may compound the length of time required to learn new tasks and may impact other aspects of rehabilitation such as social and familial adjustment. In the more severe cases, in which lingering cognitive and behavioral deficits persist, return to school and work, as well as successful social integration, can be compromised.

The clinician should also be alert to pre-injury conditions or characteristics that compromise current cognitive functioning, including prolonged substance abuse histories, prior traumatic brain injury, learning disabilities, or genetic disorders. Since the success of rehabilitation depends largely on new learning, this is an important issue.

Personality and Behavioral Issues

Most SCI individuals do not fit the "norm" in terms of psychological epidemiology. The best predictor of future behavior is still past behavior. Hence, deriving a careful history with regard to developmental, legal, psychiatric, vocational and social difficulties is most important. A disproportionate percentage of the events that cause SCI are associated with the use or misuse of legal and illegal substances. Return to substance abuse in the rehabilitation unit is usually prevented or limited by the milieu, but research suggests a high return to substance abuse post-discharge and is an issue worthy of follow up and monitoring.

Personality testing, as well as a good behavioral history, can provide excellent prognostic information about the likelihood of compliance short- and long-term with regimens that can prevent secondary complications. This kind of behavioral "red flag" is not necessarily limited to those with a clear substance abuse history.

Long-Term Issues

Many times, a parent or spouse (often a mother or wife) becomes a permanent caregiver. The individual with SCI often experiences markedly decreasing emotional distress over the first year post-injury; the caregivers, in contrast, may have markedly increased distress. This occurs as the caregivers' support system dwindles and the amount of help provided by others diminishes. Promoting respite care (formal or informal) and attending to the emotional and physical health of the caregiver is important.

Suicide, as a cause of death, is higher among persons with SCI when compared to their age-matched able-bodied counterparts. Active suicide gestures or attempts rarely occur during the acute rehabilitation admission, but are more likely to occur later as a function of lack of recovery, interpersonal difficulties, financial distress, and significant affective disorders. Substance abuse can also be a "trigger" for suicide, particularly when accompanied by diminished social support and meaningful activity on a day-to-day

basis. Suicide gestures and threats need to be taken seriously and responded to with appropriate referral to ensure safety and adequate treatment.

Many persons with SCI do not return to paid employment. The financial benefits of disability are often of sufficient magnitude to act as a disincentive to return to paid employment. For example, many individuals would lose medical benefits and reimbursement for personal care assistants if they engaged in remunerative employment. If the patient is amenable, vocational evaluations and training options should be pursued vigorously. In the absence of a desire to attempt a return to competitive employment, persons with SCI should be encouraged to pursue meaningful activities such as wheelchair sports, family activity, church work, or other avocational pursuits.

Chronic pain is an issue for a significant minority of persons with SCI. The etiology of the discomfort may be musculoskeletal or neurological, and a thorough evaluation is appropriate. However, in many cases, no clear anatomical disorder can be established, and the patient may be diagnosed with an undifferentiated chronic pain syndrome. Pain can be an avenue for medication seeking, particularly with those who have a substance abuse or prescription drug use history. Depression or anxiety can magnify the extent and impact of chronic pain. The optimal management of chronic pain requires a multidisciplinary approach. Active versus passive coping methods should also be pursued.

Role of the Psychologist

The psychologist can provide systematically derived information of help to the patient, family and staff via structured interviews and formal psychological testing. Some psychologists use a standard battery of psychological tests. Others use combinations of interviews and tests, depending on the particular referral question and problem. It is helpful to provide specific referral information to help the psychologist guide the assessment. It is also helpful to consider a standing referral order to the psychologist for all new persons with SCI. This helps destigmatize the referral process (i.e., all SCI patients are evaluated by the rehabilitation psychologist). Psychological assessment at the earliest stages of injury (i.e., ICU) may be therapeutic. Interaction with the patient during initial rehabilitation admission also facilitates contact post-discharge. It is at this juncture where family and patient coping mechanisms become most taxed.

Psychologists can provide information about personality, intellect, affect, mood, and cognition. Identifying strengths and weaknesses in these areas is essential for vocational reintegration, as well as financial and driving competency. This information can be used to guide treatment decisions and discharge plans. Assessment of problematic pre-injury behaviors, which are likely to be predictive of future difficulties, can also be accomplished. Psychological evaluation can be useful in formulating behavioral management strategies.

Psychologists participate in educational activities for persons with SCI. Educationally focused groups tend to work better than traditional group psychotherapy. Topics commonly discussed include sexuality, body image changes, disability rights, assertiveness, and family relations. Individual interventions can also be provided, ranging from stress management techniques, such as relaxation training and biofeedback, to cognitive-behavioral approaches stressing improvements in problem solving ability and coping style. Behavioral programming is sometimes necessary and can be quite effective and helpful in managing problem behaviors. This requires the cooperation of the entire staff and is an activity that requires a considerable investment of time and resources. Sex

education and counseling are important interventions, which are discussed in the next chapter. Psychologists often facilitate and coordinate peer visitation programs to assist individuals with SCI in the coping process. Timing for this intervention is critical as peer visitation is unlikely to be beneficial if the person with SCI is not receptive to the idea.

SCI has a demonstrated negative impact on romantic relationships. Physicians need to recognize developing and ongoing stressors, as well as behavioral and emotional difficulties in persons with SCI post-discharge. If marital or family difficulties are identified, the psychologist can provide expert assessment. If further counseling or therapy is required, the psychologist can organize treatment. Alternatively, care may be coordinated with other mental health professionals.

Chapter 15

Sexuality and Spinal Cord Injury

Stanley Ducharme

Introduction

With longer life expectancies following SCI, the emphasis of contemporary rehabilitation programs has gradually shifted to improving quality of life. Toward this goal, issues related to sexuality must be addressed by the rehabilitation team in both the acute and chronic stages of SCI. Providing sexual education to patients and their partners is best accomplished by an interdisciplinary team approach in which both medical and psychological issues can be addressed.

Male Sexual Act

Erectile and ejaculatory function are complex physiological activities that require interaction among the vascular, nervous and endocrine systems. Erections are controlled by the parasympathetic nervous system, whereas ejaculation is controlled by the sympathetic nervous system.

In the simplest of terms, erection is controlled by a reflex arc that is mediated in the sacral spinal cord. A reflex involves an afferent and efferent limb. The afferent limb consists of somatic afferent fibers from the genital region that travel through the pudendal nerve into the sacral spinal cord. The efferent limb involves parasympathetic fibers that originate in the sacral spinal cord. These fibers travel through the cauda equina and exit via the S2 to S4 nerve roots. The post-ganglionic parasympathetic fibers secrete nitric oxide, which causes relaxation of the smooth muscle of the corpus cavernosum and increases blood flow to the penile arteries. Consequently, the vascular sinusoids of the penis become engorged with blood, and the result is an erection. This reflex is modulated by higher brain stem, subcortical and cortical centers. In addition, erectile function is influenced by hormonal factors such as testosterone.

Ejaculation signals the culmination of the male sexual act and is primarily controlled by the sympathetic nervous system. Similar to the sympathetic innervation of the bladder, these fibers originate in the thoraco-lumbar spinal cord and travel into the sympathetic chain. These fascicles then travel through the splanchnic nerves into the hypogastric plexus. After synapsing in the inferior mesenteric ganglion, postganglionic fibers travel through the hypogastric nerves to supply the vas deferens, seminal vesicles and ejaculatory ducts in the prostate.

Female Sexual Act

The physiology of the female sexual act has not been studied as well as the male sexual act. However, female sexual satisfaction is dependent on a complex interaction of the endocrine and nervous systems. Sexual excitation is the result of psychogenic and

physical stimulation. This arousal is manifested by vaginal lubrication and tightening of the introitus. Stimulation of the genital region, including the clitoris, labia majora, and labia minora, causes afferent signals to travel via the pudendal nerve into the S2 to S4 segments of the spinal cord. These fibers interact with efferent parasympathetic fibers that project through the pelvic nerve. The result is dilation of arteries to perineal muscles and tightening of the introitus. In addition, the parasympathetic fibers cause the Bartholin's glands to secrete mucus, which aids in vaginal lubrication.

Female orgasm is characterized by the rhythmic contraction of the pelvic structures. Female orgasm also results in cervical dilation, which may aid in sperm transport and fertility.

Sexual History

A simplified sexual history should be part of the initial clinical assessment. Key elements include physical capabilities, past sexual activities, and current sexual function. In addition, the clinician should inquire into partner availability, partner satisfaction, sexual orientation, behavioral repertoire, and past sexual abuse. Open-ended questions will facilitate better communication. Topics of a more sensitive nature should be reserved for later in the interview, when a therapeutic relationship has been established.

Psychological Considerations

Adaptation to an SCI is a gradual process that extends over a prolonged period of time. Successful sexual adjustment is influenced by many factors such as age at time of injury, quality of social supports, physical health, gender, and severity of the injury. Losses need to be mourned so that the remaining strengths can be nurtured and developed. To achieve satisfying sexual adjustment, a person with an SCI will have to learn to value their new sexual abilities, as opposed to recapturing the past.

After a traumatic injury, individuals typically go through a period of reduced sexual drive. Although libido is not affected by SCI, it may be diminished by depression, trauma of the injury, or medications. Initially after injury some persons with SCI may deny the importance of sexual issues. Other individuals may be reluctant to discuss issues related to sexuality due to cultural or personal reasons. Other patients may go through a period of sexual "acting out" (i.e., unacceptable sexually explicit language, inappropriate unwanted physical contact with staff, etc.) while on the rehabilitation unit.

During the acute rehabilitation phase, a sensitive discussion regarding sexuality is appropriate. The person with SCI may inquire about issues such as dating, attractiveness, relationships, parenthood and physical appearance. Other topics of interest many include erections, lubrication, sensation, orgasm, ejaculation and fertility. Many individuals will inquire about sexuality as it relates to bladder and bowel function. Even if the patient does not initiate discussion about these topics, it is important for members of the rehabilitation team to provide basic information.

Male and Female Arousal

Men and women with SCI often lack sensation at traditional erogenous areas such as the genitals and nipples. As such, stimulating these areas may result in penile erections or vaginal lubrication, but not necessarily sexual pleasure. However, other areas, sometimes not normally recognized as erogenous areas, such as the ears, eyelids and neck, can be

stimulated to provide sexual arousal. Some individuals find the skin surfaces around the neurological level to have heightened tactile sexual response.

Male Sexual Function: Erections, Ejaculation and Orgasm

Men with SCI may obtain reflexogenic or psychogenic erections. Reflex erections are secondary to manual stimulation of the genital region. Psychogenic erections are the result of erotic stimuli that result in cortical modulation of the sacral reflex arc. In general, erections are more likely with incomplete injuries (both upper and lower motor neuron), than complete injuries. Many times, men with SCI can only maintain an erection while the penis is stimulated, and the quality of the erection is insufficient for sexual satisfaction. As such, the erection must be augmented with devices, medications or a penile implant for satisfactory sexual function.

In men with SCI, the ability to ejaculate is less common than the ability to obtain an erection. The rate of ejaculation varies depending on the location and nature of the neurological injury. In complete upper motor neuron lesions, the ejaculation rate is estimated at 2 percent. In incomplete upper motor neuron lesions, the ejaculation rate is estimated to be somewhat higher at 32 percent. Many men who are able to ejaculate experience retrograde ejaculation into the bladder; some may experience dribbling of semen.

The experience of orgasm in men with SCI is variable. Some individuals describe a primarily emotional event. Others experience generalized muscle relaxation or a pleasurable sensation in the pelvis or at the sensory level. Other men report orgasm to be non-existent following the injury.

Oral Therapy for Male Sexual Dysfunction

Sildenafil (Viagra), vardenafil (Levitra), and tadalafil (Cialis) are phosphodiesterase type 5 inhibitors. This class of drugs prevents intracorporeal breakdown of cyclic GNP. Phosphodiesterase type 5 inhibitors are rapidly absorbed after oral administration and are taken approximately 60 minutes before anticipated sexual activity. They are most effective for men who are capable of achieving reflex erections and can assist the man in gaining further rigidity and in sustaining the erection for penetration. These medications are contraindicated in men taking nitrates due to the risk of profound hypotension. Many men with SCI have low baseline blood pressures, and this agent should be prescribed with caution. In addition, this drug is not recommended for those individuals with cardiac disease. Other side effects include facial flushing, dyspepsia, headache and visual disturbances. Oral therapy has supplanted other treatment strategies; intracavernosal and transurethral therapy and penile vacuum devices are less utilized in contemporary clinical practice.

Intracavernosal Injection Therapy

Therapy with intracavernosal injection (Figure 15.1) of papaverine, alprostadil, and phentolamine is an accepted treatment of erectile dysfunction. Initiating this therapy necessitates a referral to a urologist. Initially, individuals are given small doses of the pharmacological agent, and the dose is increased until a satisfactory erection is obtained

Figure 15.1
Intracavernosal Injection Therapy

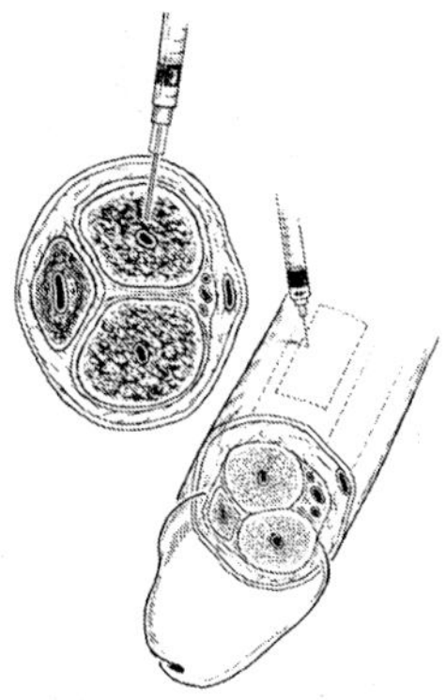

for intercourse. Sometimes, a mixture of agents is prescribed. Erections should not persist beyond four hours. Many tetraplegics have impaired hand function and will require a cooperative partner to perform the injection. In some cases, a commercially marketed penile autoinjector can be easier to manipulate. Priapism is a possibility; therefore, both partners should be properly trained. Some individuals with incomplete injuries may experience pain at the injection site. Penile fibrosis is also a potential risk of intracavernosal therapy.

Transurethral Therapy

Transurethral delivery systems for administering agents that result in erections are available. The medication delivered is usually alprostadil. This treatment is generally not as effective as intracavernosal therapy. Many men are not satisfied with the rigidity of the erections obtained.

Penile Vacuum Devices

These devices create a vacuum around the penis (Figure 15.2). As a result, blood is drawn into the corporal spaces. A band is then slipped off the plastic cylinder around the base of the penis to maintain penile tumescence. Ejaculation may be retarded due to the constriction of the urethra. However, newer models are available with constricting bands that are less likely to diminish ejaculation.

Vacuum devices are non-invasive, economical and efficacious. However, these devices require some degree of manual dexterity. For many men with tetraplegia, the partner must be willing to assist with the procedure. In addition, men must transfer out of the wheelchair and be in a recumbent position to obtain a good vacuum seal at the base of the penis. Individuals with incomplete injuries may experience pain, discoloration, and coldness at the penis. Constriction rings should not remain in place for more than 30 minutes. Longer time periods may be associated with potential skin breakdown. Vacuum devices are more accepted by men in more established sexual relationships. Some men use vacuum devices to augment erections obtained with oral medications. Vacuum devices are commonly used in developing nations where pharmacotherapy is unavailable or not affordable.

Figure 15.2
Penile Vacuum Device

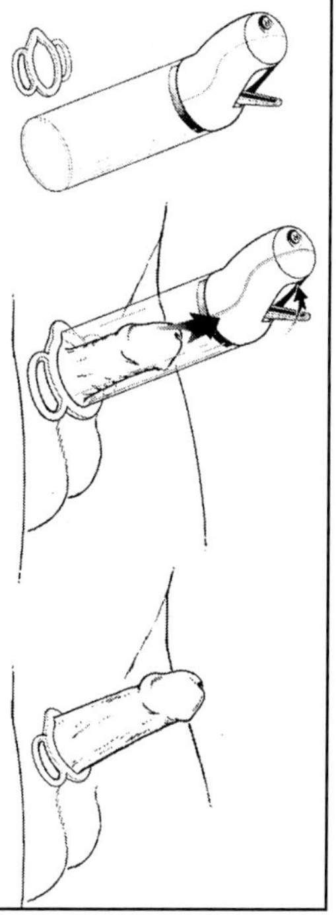

Penile Implants

Penile implants are considered when other treatments have been unsuccessful, especially if trauma has disrupted the penile vascular system. It also may be indicated if severe Peyronie's disease is a factor. Implants are not considered in the first year post-injury so that persons with SCI can make emotional adaptations to the injury and explore less invasive options for sexual activity. There are a number of different devices, ranging from the simple malleable prosthesis to more complex hydraulic prostheses. Generally, the choice of prosthesis is related to individual preference and financial constraints.

Figure 15.3 **Penile Vibroejaculator**

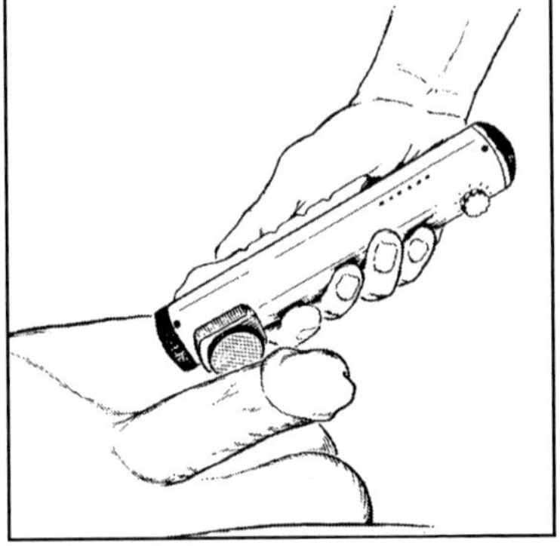

Male Fertility

The ability to father a child correlates with the frequency of ejaculation. Successful pregnancy rates range from 10 percent to 35 percent. In general, men with incomplete lesions (both upper and lower motor neuron) are more likely to become fathers than are those with complete lesions. Conditions that may contribute to infertility include retrograde ejaculation, repeated urinary tract infections, and altered testicular temperature. Newer methods of obtaining semen samples include rectal electroejaculation or penile vibroejaculation (Figure 15.3). Both of these techniques may precipitate autonomic dysreflexia.

Female Sexual Function: Sexual Arousal and Vaginal Lubrication

Most women with SCI can achieve some level of vaginal lubrication. This lubrication can be mediated by reflexogenic or psychogenic factors. Individuals with incomplete (both upper and lower motor neuron) injuries are more likely to have satisfactory lubrication. If vaginal lubrication is unsatisfactory, then a water soluble lubricant can be recommended. Sildenafil may be of value in women with SCI by increasing blood flow to the perineum, and increasing vaginal lubrication, which may improve sexual satisfaction. However, there are no controlled studies on the female SCI population.

Female Fertility

Immediately after injury, 44 percent to 58 percent of women suffer from temporary amenorrhea. Menstruation usually returns within six months post-injury. Neither the level nor the completeness of the injury appear to be associated with interruption of menstrual cycles. In a small percentage of women with SCI, there are also changes in cycle length, duration of flow, amount of flow, and amount of menstrual pain. Most women with SCI are fertile.

Contraception

Most menstruating women with spinal cord injury are fertile. In this context, an open dialogue regarding contraception is essential. Condoms provide contraception, as well as

diminish the risk of transmission of sexually transmitted diseases. A diaphragm may be another acceptable option if the individual has adequate hand dexterity or a cooperative partner. Oral contraception is associated with increased incidence of thromboembolism, and must be prescribed with caution in women with SCI. Oral contraceptives that contain only progesterone may be safer than medications that contain both estrogen and progesterone. IUD may be associated with increased incidence of pelvic inflammatory disease. Untreated PID may lead to autonomic dysreflexia. In addition, women with SCI may not be able to perceive if the device has migrated out of the cervix.

Pregnancy

Pregnant women with SCI have an increased risk of urinary tract infections, leg edema, autonomic dysreflexia, constipation, thromboembolism and premature birth. Since uterine innervation arises from the T10 to T12 levels, patients with lesions above T10 may not be able to perceive uterine contractions or fetal movements. It may be difficult to differentiate between pregnancy induced hypertension (pre-eclampsia) and autonomic dysreflexia. Autonomic dysreflexia may be the only clinical manifestation of labor. During the second and third trimester, pregnant women may have difficulties in performing functional tasks that were previously completed independently. Transfers may require the assistance of a caregiver, and a power wheelchair may be necessary for mobility. Locating an obstetrician and anesthesiologist with a supportive attitude, an accessible office, and experience in SCI can be difficult in many areas.

Urinary and Fecal Incontinence

Urinary and fecal incontinence at inopportune times and subsequent social rejection are major fears of some people with SCI. A bladder or bowel accident may occur at any time during courtship, sexual activity, or during social events. The embarrassment, shame, and humiliation associated with incontinence create undue anxiety and are often regarded as a major reason for social isolation or the termination of a relationship.

To minimize untimely episodes of incontinence, the bladder should be emptied prior to sexual activity. Foley catheters, if present, can be taped to the side of the penis with a condom placed over the catheter. Females can engage in sexual intercourse despite the presence of a Foley catheter by taping the catheter to the abdomen. Despite the best management program, sexual stimulation can cause urinary and/or fecal incontinence. Embarrassing passage of gas from the vagina, bowel or ostomy bag can be avoided by gentle thrusting, coital positioning, and a careful diet. Fluids should be limited during the hours preceding sexual activity. Towels should be available to manage episodes of urinary or fecal incontinence.

Conclusion

Sexual adaptation after an SCI is a gradual process that involves psychological and physical adjustments. The availability of medications, devices and procedures have greatly enhanced the possibility of having a satisfactory sexual life after an SCI. Toward this end, the rehabilitation team has a responsibility to provide sexual information and counseling during the acute and chronic stages of SCI.

Chapter 16

Aging and Spinal Cord Injury

Elizabeth Roaf

Introduction

The care of patients with long-term SCI is a challenging and rewarding task. Optimal care of this population requires an understanding of both the rehabilitation and medical issues. Of equal importance is an appreciation of the physiology of aging. People with chronic SCI suffer from many of the same medical disorders as neurologically intact individuals. The clinical manifestations of these medical conditions, however, may be atypical (e.g., age of onset, signs and symptoms) due to the complex physiologic changes associated with SCI. Therefore, every person with an SCI should have a skilled primary care physician; this practitioner may be an internist, physiatrist or family physician.

The Aging Lung

Prior to considering the effects of chronic SCI on lung function, the effects of aging must be understood. Vital capacity (total exhalation after a maximal inspiration) normally peaks at approximately age 20, then gradually diminishes by 1 percent per year. Although vital capacity decreases with age, total lung capacity does not. Thus, the residual volume of the lung increases as the vital capacity diminishes. The loss of vital capacity may occur due to lack of deep-breathing activities as older adults frequently become more sedentary. Vital capacity also diminishes acutely with lung infections and mucus plugging. Patients with baseline reduced vital capacities and tidal volumes who do not take occasional deep breaths can rapidly develop collapse of the small airways and alveoli (microatelectasis). In addition, the elastic recoil of the lung diminishes with aging. Microatelectasis, with concomitant diminished lung capacity, may result in non-uniform ventilation, especially in the dependent portions of the lung.

Cough may be weakened due to age-related changes in lung mechanics, as well as decreased intercostal and abdominal muscle strength. Weakened cough impacts secretion clearance and may prolong the course of respiratory infections.

Pulmonary Diseases in Chronic SCI

Pulmonary diseases are major sources of morbidity and mortality in SCI. By some estimates, respiratory illnesses (i.e., pneumonia and bronchitis) are the leading cause of mortality in long-term SCI patients. Tetraplegics and high-level paraplegics have impaired cough mechanisms due to paralysis of the abdominal and intercostal muscles. These patients have difficulty clearing secretions and are at high risk for pneumonia.

Treatment of an SCI patient with an acute respiratory infection includes the standard approach to ill individuals with respiratory disease (i.e., history, physical examination, complete blood count, blood cultures, chest X-ray, sputum analysis, antibiotics, etc.).

Loosening of secretions should be attempted with warm mist via tracheostomy mask or half face mask. Nebulizer treatment with albuterol may be needed. Inhaled, oral or intravenous steroids may be indicated. As SCI patients have impaired pulmonary mechanics, intubation may be required.

Beyond these standard approaches, individuals with chronic SCI may need aggressive physical therapy interventions, including frequent suctioning, chest percussion, postural drainage, and assisted cough ("quad cough"). These treatments can be provided by the respiratory or physical therapy services. The frequency of these interventions should be individualized, but, in some cases, therapy is required every two hours. Oxygen saturation should be monitored frequently, and arterial blood gas (ABG) measurement should be done in patients with a known history of carbon dioxide retention or those who appear to be fatiguing.

If ventilation appears to be a necessary intervention, noninvasive positive pressure ventilation should be considered. Generally administered by a mask that fits over the nose, noninvasive positive pressure ventilation may be either continuous (CPAP) or bilevel (BIPAP). Although these methods are generally used for chronic hypoventilation syndromes, short periods of CPAP and aggressive secretion management may prevent intubation in an acute crisis. This should be considered in individuals with high-level lesions in which extubation may be challenging.

Individuals with long-term disability have often had multiple different courses of antibiotics and may have strains of bacteria that are highly resistant to many antibiotics. Patients with tracheostomies may be colonized with pseudomonas, which can make analysis of sputum (colonization vs. infection) complex. Infectious disease consultation may be warranted in such cases.

Global Alveolar Hypoventilation

Global alveolar hypoventilation (GAH) is an insidious, restrictive process that may compromise pulmonary function in SCI patients. GAH is an ongoing, subclinical loss of ventilatory function due to loss of pulmonary compliance from chronic hypoventilation or scarring. This condition can lead to progressive respiratory failure and subsequent need for long-term ventilation. Chronically, it may be exacerbated by obesity, kyphosis and scoliosis. Subclinical hypercapnia and sleep disorders may also exacerbate GAH. Symptoms of worsening restrictive lung disease include nightmares, morning headaches, daytime drowsiness, dyspnea on exertion, orthopnea, and generalized fatigue. Caregivers may note paradoxical breathing.

Assessment of lung function should be a part of routine health-care maintenance, especially in those patients with complete high cervical lesions. Surveillance of lung function should include periodic arterial blood gas measurement to assess the degree, if any, of carbon dioxide retention. In addition to arterial blood gas monitoring, pulmonary function testing should be ordered every few years in tetraplegic individuals and some at-risk high-level paraplegics.

Chronic ventilation may become necessary to sustain life in some individuals who develop chronic hypoventilation. Ventilation may be invasive or noninvasive. The most common types of noninvasive positive pressure ventilation used are CPAP and BIPAP, which are often administered nasally via mask. Alternatives to CPAP and BIPAP include intermittent positive pressure ventilation (IPPV) via mouthpiece and negative pressure

ventilators (e.g., raincoat, cuirass and mini iron lung). IPPV may initially be prescribed for episodic use throughout the day to maintain adequate carbon dioxide exchange. The raincoat ventilation device covers the thorax and has long sleeves that allow for a tight seal to the body. The cuirass ventilator is a hard shell-shaped device that fits over the chest. A tube (similar in appearance to a vacuum cleaner hose) is connected to the device which causes negative pressure and facilitates ventilation. The mini iron lung is a more compact version of the iron lung used in the past to treat polio. Successful negative pressure ventilation requires a small body habitus without significant kyphosis and scoliosis.

Cardiac Disorders

Coronary heart disease is the leading cause of death in adults in the United States. As life expectancy of individuals with SCI has increased, mortality from coronary artery disease has increased. Risk factors include elevated total serum cholesterol, increased low-density lipoprotein, depressed high-density lipoprotein, obesity, family history of heart disease, diabetes, smoking, hypertension and immobility. Individuals with SCI may be at increased risk for CAD due to relative inactivity, insulin insensitivity or diminished HDL levels. The wide variations in blood pressure from autonomic instability secondary to SCI may cause intimal damage.

In tetraplegia and high-level paraplegia, pain perception is impaired due to disruption of spinal afferent pathways from the heart and coronary vessels. This disruption is less profound in incomplete lesions. Nociception may be further impaired by coexisting medical conditions (e.g., diabetes with autonomic neuropathy). Cardiac ischemia and infarctions may present with unusual pain referral patterns, symptoms of autonomic dysreflexia, or other atypical presentations. Silent ischemia and infarction are also a possibility.

Screening for heart disease begins with a thorough clinical assessment. Risk factors should be identified. However, physical exam findings must be interpreted with caution. For example, chronic peripheral edema may be due to dependency and lack of muscle tone, and not secondary to right heart failure. Auscultation of the lungs may reveal crackles that may be secondary to left heart failure. Alternatively, these findings may be secondary to pulmonary scarring and atelectasis.

Investigations to evaluate ischemic heart disease may include arm ergometry exercise testing in paraplegics or low-level tetraplegics. Persantine thallium or MIBI studies may also be helpful. Since standard cardiac stress tests are not as diagnostically valuable in women, a dolbutamine echocardiography should be considered. This test is also useful in those individuals who cannot perform upper arm ergometry.

In SCI patients, echocardiography may show atrophy of cardiac musculature in a symmetric fashion. The symmetrical atrophy is most likely due to lack of cardiac loading from immobility, profound orthostatic hypotension, and diminished venous return. These echocardiographic abnormalities are different from the concentric cardiac hypertrophy seen in able-bodied patients with hypertension.

SCI patients with CAD should be managed in similar fashion to other patients. Modifiable risk factors should be addressed. The spectrum of interventions available to able-bodied patients should be offered to SCI patients (i.e., lifestyle changes, medications, angioplasty and CABG).

Introduction of medications should be done cautiously as many patients with SCI have low baseline blood pressures and, consequently, may not be able to tolerate traditional doses of anti-anginal medications.

Osteoporosis

Osteoporosis is a group of disorders affecting bone, characterized by decreased osteoblastic formation relative to osteoclastic resorption. This results in a net loss of bone. Osteoporosis may be generalized or localized.

Following an acute SCI, patients suffer from regional osteoporosis syndrome. Twenty to 50 percent of bone mass in lower extremities is lost within the first few months. Bone mobilization may occur beginning as early as the first two weeks following injury. More typically, bone resorption begins around week four to five post-injury. Peak mobilization is at approximately the 16th week post-injury. The mobilization of calcium gradually diminishes and reaches a plateau between five to 24 months post-injury. This is due to both increased osteoclastic activity post-injury and decreased osteoblastic activity. Most patients will experience hypercalciuria and hydroxyprolinuria.

Some male patients with acute cervical lesions may develop clinically significant hypercalcemia secondary to osteoporosis. Symptoms of hypercalcemia may include nausea, vomiting, malaise, anorexia, headache, gastric distention, abdominal pain, fecal impaction and depression. With severe hypercalcemia, seizures, cardiac arrhythmia and death are possible. Treatment of hypercalcemia begins with hydration with normal saline solution followed by diuresis with furosemide. Treatment bisphosphonates (etidronate, alendronate) may be needed in refractory cases. If the hypercalcemia is severe (symptoms of cardiac or CNS impairment) management should be in an intensive care unit.

Osteoporosis is defined as bone density less than or equal to 2.5 standard deviations from the mean on bone densitometry evaluation. Laboratory evaluation of osteoporosis should include measurement of serum calcium (to rule out bony metastases), phosphorus, parathormone (PTH, elevated in hyperparathyroidism), and serum alkaline phosphatase. Serum levels of calcium, phosphorus, alkaline phosphatase and PTH should be normal in individuals with osteoporosis. Individuals with SCI should be screened yearly for hyperthyroidism (TSH, T4 levels) since this is a treatable cause of osteoporosis.

There is an increased risk of fractures from profound disuse osteoporosis in SCI. Paraplegics will develop osteoporosis in the lower extremities. Quadriplegics also develop osteoporosis in the distal upper extremities. However, SCI is not associated with osteoporosis in the spine. Osteoporotic fractures may occur as early as a few years post-injury. The risk of osteoporosis may be lower in individuals with significant spasticity in their limbs; moderate to severe spastic muscles may exert forces on bone and decrease bone resorption.

Femur fractures are commonly encountered osteoporotic fractures in long-term SCI patients. They may occur subsequent to significant trauma such as a fall. However, minor trauma associated with transfers or PROM exercises may precipitate a fracture. This condition may present with pain, increased spasticity, swelling, erythema, autonomic dysreflexia or even low-grade fevers. With any fracture, orthopedic consultation is essential. Many times, femur fractures in SCI patients are managed non-operatively. Malunion and nonunion should be avoided. Malunion can lead to impaired sitting. As a result, patients may develop pressure ulcers and contractures. Impaired sitting can also

lead to pelvic obliquity and scoliosis.

Slowing the progression of osteoporosis is essential. Although the literature is replete with information regarding interventions for prevention and treatment in the otherwise healthy population, the literature on safe, appropriate, effective treatment of osteoporosis for individuals with SCI is inadequate. Individuals with hypovitaminosis D, not reaching the level of vitamin D deficiency, may be supplemented with oral vitamin D 2,000 IU per day. Consultation with an endocrinologist is appropriate. Supplementation with vitamin D 50,000 IU weekly for six to eight weeks may be indicated. Calcium supplementation is controversial in persons with SCI due to the increased risk of developing kidney and bladder stones. In individuals with long-term SCI, screening bone densitometry may be indicated. In selected patients, a trial of a bisphosphonate (i.e., Fosamax) or calcitonin, in addition to vitamin D, should be considered.

Musculoskeletal Pain

The incidence of chronic pain in the SCI population is estimated between 20 percent and 50 percent. Pain may be musculoskeletal, neuropathic or visceral in origin.

Upper extremity pain is common. People with SCI load joints that do not normally bear weight (i.e., shoulder, elbow and wrist). This predisposes them to painful upper extremity conditions. Symptoms of upper extremity pain, dysesthesias or weakness should be evaluated thoroughly. Due to impaired sensation, SCI patients may have atypical presentations of common disorders. Rotator cuff tendonitis, rotator cuff tears, subacromial bursitis, cervical radiculopathy, carpal tunnel syndrome, lateral epicondylitis, medial epicondylitis, and myofascial pain are potential pathologic entities. Rotator cuff tendonitis is common and often slow in response to treatment, due to overuse of the upper extremities. Relative rest of the affected extremities, NSAIDS and icing are the first-line treatment. Steroid injection may be indicated. Less common causes of upper extremity discomfort include syringomyelia, heterotopic ossification, angina, aortic dissection and Pancoast tumors.

When prescribing a treatment plan, however, a few special issues must be addressed. The shoulder of an SCI individual is synonymous with the hip of an able-bodied person. Therefore, shoulder pain in the SCI population may have significant functional consequences. Transfers that could previously be performed independently may now require the assistance of a caregiver. If absolute or relative rest is required, a patient who was previously using a manual wheelchair may be temporarily required to use a power wheelchair. Modalities, such as ice, hot packs and ultrasound, must be prescribed with caution due to impaired sensation. Surgery for a completely torn rotator cuff tendon puts the patient at risk for secondary complications, including pressure ulcers.

Neuropathic Pain

Neuropathic pain may be of central or peripheral origin. Patients will complain of a burning, shooting or lancing pain. The discomfort may involve the abdomen, rectum or lower extremities. It may be exacerbated by other noxious stimuli, including urinary tract infections, renal stones, HO, etc. Neuropathic pain is more common with incomplete lesions.

Neuropathic pain requires a complete assessment. Structural anatomical pathology that may be contributing to the discomfort should be identified and, if possible, treated

(i.e., syrinx formation, nephrolithiasis, etc.). Although neuropathic pain is not usually responsive to acetaminophen or nonsteroidal anti-inflammatory drugs, a short trial of these medications is not unreasonable. Although frequently prescribed for neuropathic pain, tricyclic antidepressants (TCA), such as amitriptyline, imipramine and nortriptyline, should be used with caution in patients with SCI (Table 1). Tricyclic antidepressants have dose-dependent, anti-cholinergic side effects that may cause urinary retention, dry mouth, blurred vision, and orthostatic hypotension. In individuals with baseline orthostatic hypotension and urinary retention, these side effects may be significant. Before instituting therapy with a TCA, an EKG to exclude conduction defects should be completed. Anti-seizure medications, such as carbamazepine (Tegretol) and gabapentin (Neurontin), can be considered to palliate neuropathic pain in individuals with SCI. In cases of refractory pain, a trial of baclofen, titrating up to 15 mg tid, may help alleviate pain symptoms. Monitoring of liver function tests is required while on baclofen.

Table 1
Medications to Treat Neuropathic Pain

Medication	Brand Name	Starting Dose	Maximum Dose	Precautions
amitriptyline	Elavil	10-25 mg qhs	150 mg qhs	anticholinergic
nortriptyline	Pamelor	10-25 mg qhs	150 mg qhs	anticholinergic
imipramine	Tofranil	10-25 mg qhs	150 mg qhs	less anticholinergic
carbamazepine	Tegretol	200 mg bid	400 mg qid	agranulocytosis, thrombocytopenia, sedation, dizziness; monitor drug levels
gabapentin	Neurontin	100 mg tid	900 mg po tid	sedation, ataxia, diplopia; renal dose adjustments
pregabalin	Lyrica	50 mg tid	300 mg/day	abrupt withdrawal renal dose adjustment depression alcohol use CHF class III or IV
duloxetine	Cymbalta	30 mg qd	60 mg/day	renal dosing hepatic dosing suicidality in children/ young adults schizophrenia in the elderly hypertension
doxepin	Silenor	10 mg qd	300 mg/day	suicidality in young adults acute MI cardiac disease urinary retention elderly diabetes mellitus Parkinson's seizure disorder

Syringomyelia

Post-traumatic syringomyelia is a complication of SCI that may result in functional loss. This phenomenon affects approximately 5 percent of those with SCI. The incidence of syrinx may be slightly higher with tetraplegia vs. paraplegia. Syringomyelia may be recognized in acute or chronic phases of SCI. Many patients with syringomyelia, however, do not have any clinically recognizable signs or symptoms.

The pathogenesis of post-traumatic syringomyelia is not entirely understood. Cavitation of the spinal cord usually occurs at the level of the initial injury. Cavity formation may be secondary to liquefaction of the spinal cord or from the central hematoma present at the initial injury. Adhesions from arachnoiditis may exacerbate the cavity formation. The lesion usually progresses in a cephalad direction. As the lesion progresses and compromises more nerve fibers, symptoms may become more apparent. Rarely, a syrinx may extend from the cervical spinal cord into the brain stem.

Potential symptoms include increased pain and spasticity. Dysautonomic features may also be identified, such as new onset orthostatic hypotension or frank autonomic dysreflexia. In addition, some patients will experience progressive weakness, dysesthesias and hyperhidrosis. Trigeminal nerve deficit and Horner's syndrome may present if the syrinx extends into the upper cervical segments. If the lesion involves the brain stem, manifestations include hiccups, nystagmus, recurrent laryngeal nerve palsy, or death. Syringomyelia-related symptoms may be exacerbated by coughing, sneezing or body movement.

A post-traumatic syringomyelia is best visualized with gadolinium enhanced magnetic resonance imaging study. Radiological findings include decreased signal intensity on T1 weighted images and enhancement of the cyst. Other radiological findings include arachnoiditis, adhesions and gliosis.

Treatment of asymptomatic syringomyelia consists of regular surveillance of the neurological level and serial MRI studies. Surgical intervention with percutaneous drainage of the cavity or shunting of the CSF into the subarachnoid space or peritoneum may be warranted in progressive symptomatic cases. Surgical interventions may be of limited success as loculated cysts can be difficult to effectively drain and shunts may become blocked or infected. Either of these two scenarios may lead to a recurrence of syringomyelia formation.

Abdominal Disorders

Evaluation of abdominal pathology in SCI patients with potentially impaired sensation can be very difficult. The typical clinical features of the acute abdomen, such as fever, guarding and rebound, may be absent. Pain, when present, may be atypical in quality and location.

Increased spasticity and a general feeling of unwellness may be the only manifestations of a surgical emergency. Cholecystitis, pancreatitis, appendicitis, gastric and duodenal ulcers, abdominal malignancies, and volvulus are some of the diagnostic possibilities. Urological causes must also be considered, including nephrolithiasis, epididymitis and testicular torsion. Urological pathology, including bladder stones and bladder cancer, should also be considered. Patients with repeated urinary tract infections or indwelling catheters have higher rates of squamous cell cancers of the bladder, an aggressive form of bladder cancer. In women, gynecological pathology, such as ectopic

pregnancy, ruptured ovarian cysts, or pelvic inflammatory diseases, can result in an acute abdomen.

When warranted, consultation with the appropriate surgical service should be obtained promptly. Not all surgical consultants have experience with SCI patients, and rehabilitation physicians may, on occasion, be required to advocate for necessary evaluations, investigations and treatments.

Hepatitis

Individuals with chronic SCI may be at increased risk for hepatitis B and C, if they were injured before 1992 and received blood products. Other risk factors include a history of intravenous drug use, multiple sexual partners, and HIV infection. In Asian-Americans, rates of hepatitis B are high. The virus is known to be transmitted by pregnant women to their children (i.e., vertical transmission). Hepatitis C is being increasingly detected. Transmission may be from household exposure. Screening for hepatitis B and C exposure is reasonable. Patients with hepatitis should be referred to a gastroenterologist for further evaluation and treatment.

Venous Thromboembolism

The risk of venous thromboembolism (VTE) is low in healthy individuals with chronic SCI. VTE prophylaxis, such as low molecular weight heparin, should be considered during periods of hospitalization or prolonged illness.

Chapter 17

Wheelchair Mobility

Amy Bjornson

For most people with an SCI, a wheelchair is essential for independent mobility. In some cases, individuals may ambulate with an assistive device indoors (i.e., Canadian forearm crutches) and use a wheelchair for community mobility. Others may use a manual wheelchair (Figure 17.1) for short distances and a power wheelchair (Figure 17.4) for longer distances. Furthermore, some individuals may own two wheelchairs: one for athletic pursuits (i.e., sports wheelchair) and a wheelchair for daily activities. It is imperative to understand that, in many cases, individuals are not confined to, but liberated by, a wheelchair. Prior to prescribing this intervention, however, a thorough wheelchair assessment must be completed. Optimal wheelchair fitting requires the close cooperation of all members of the rehabilitation team.

Figure 17.1 **Manual Wheelchair**

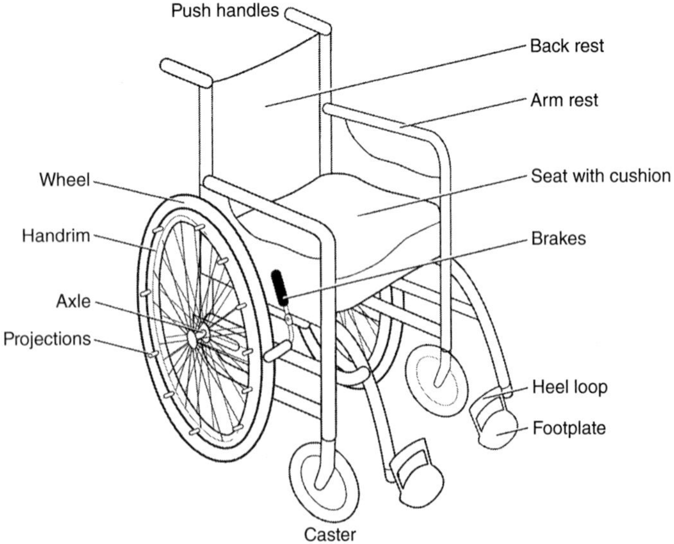

A wheelchair and seating system must maximize function. A properly fitted system will optimize upper extremity function and distribute seating pressure to minimize

the risk of pressure ulcers. In addition, proper wheelchair fitting will minimize pelvic obliquity and concomitant scoliosis and kyphosis.

Figure 17.2
Adjusting Axle Position

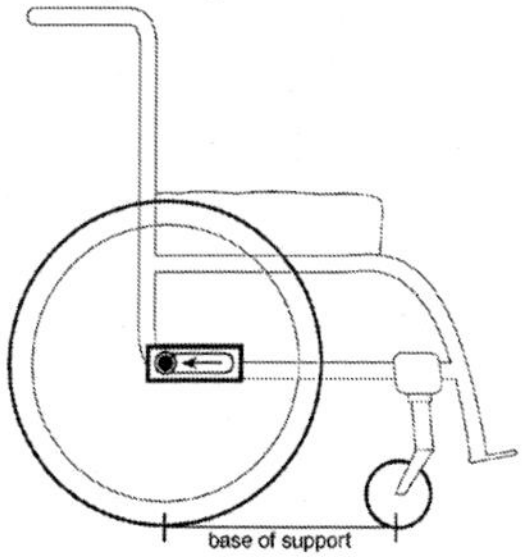

Posterior Wheel Position
Increases Stability

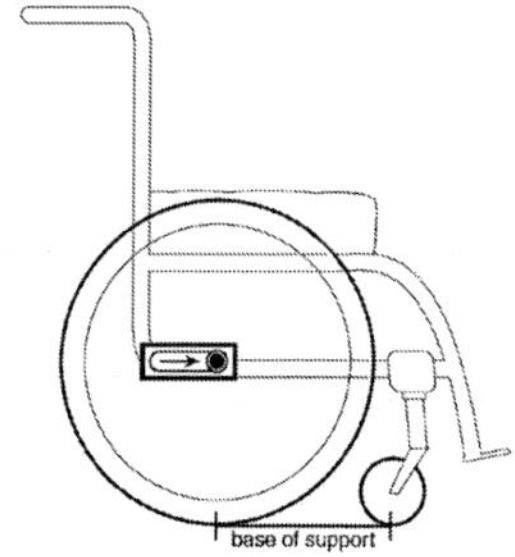

Anterior Wheel Position
Increases Manueverabilty

Types of Wheelchairs

Wheelchairs can be self-propelled (power) or propelled by the occupant (manual). Manual wheelchairs can have rigid or folding frames. Folding wheelchairs, when compared to rigid wheelchairs, are smaller, easier to transport, and less expensive. However, folding wheelchairs are heavier, less durable, and probably less energy efficient. Folding wheelchairs have more moving parts and require more frequent adjustments.

Adjusting Axle Position

By moving the wheel axle interiorly (i.e., closer to the casters), maneuverability is increased; however, this results in decreased stability by narrowing the base of support (Figure 17.2).

Seat Height

Appropriate seat height can make transfers easier. In general, it is easiest to transfer between surfaces of similar height. Lower seat heights may allow some patients to propel their wheelchair with leg movement when the upper extremities are paralyzed. Lower seat heights will also allow for easier access under tables and desks.

Figure 17.3
Tilt Angle

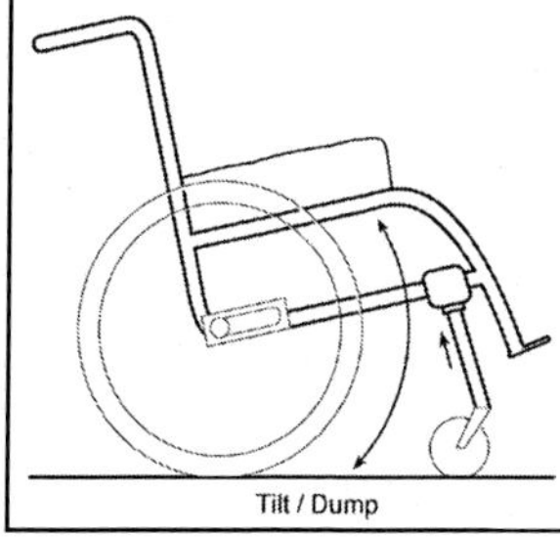

Tilt and Recline

Tilt refers to movement of the seating surface relative to the floor. With tilt adjustments, however, the angle between the seat and back remain constant (i.e., no change in back angle). Increasing the "dump" is synonymous with increasing the amount of tilt. Back angle (i.e., recline) refers to the angle between the seat and back (Figure 17.3). This angle can be adjusted to accommodate patient comfort, tone, stability and function in addition to joint range of movement.

Many power wheelchairs are equipped with power tilt and recline, which allow for pressure relief. Power recline is convenient for certain self-care tasks such as intermittent catheterization. Reclining, however, may result in shear forces that can contribute to pressure ulcers. Reclining can increase spasticity in some patients, as well.

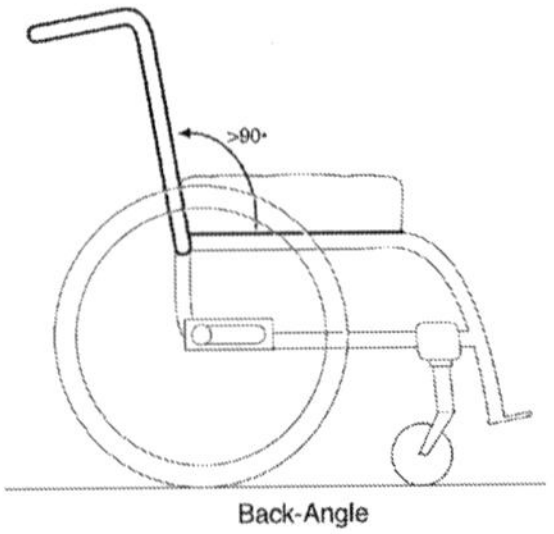

Figure 17.3
Back Angle

Leg Rests

Adjustable leg rests are essential. Many individuals will have dependent edema that will be palliated by raising the legs. Proper lower extremity support will assist in optimal weight distribution in the buttocks and thighs. If paralyzed legs are not secured, injury may result during wheelchair mobility.

Control Mechanisms for Power Wheelchairs

Joystick: the patient uses his hand to move the joystick for wheelchair control

Head control: a specialized headrest allows the patient to drive the wheelchair with movement of the head; this is useful for high tetraplegics

Chin control: a mini joystick, which is used to steer the wheelchair, is mounted in front of the patient's chin; this is also useful for high tetraplegics

Sip-and-puff: the patient pushes air through a straw, allowing for control of the wheelchair and, possibly, an environment control unit; this type of device is useful for very high tetraplegics who may not have adequate neck strength to manage a head control

Wheelchair Prescription Guidelines Based on Motor Level

High Tetraplegia (C2 to C4)

- Power wheelchair with power tilt and/or recline
- If ventilator dependent, ventilator tray
- Control system depending on functional capabilities (i.e., sip-and-puff, chin control, head control)
- Excellent pressure relief seat cushion
- High-back seat, headrest, trunk supports
- Upper extremity support such as lap board, or arm trough

Figure 17.4 **Typical Power Wheelchair**

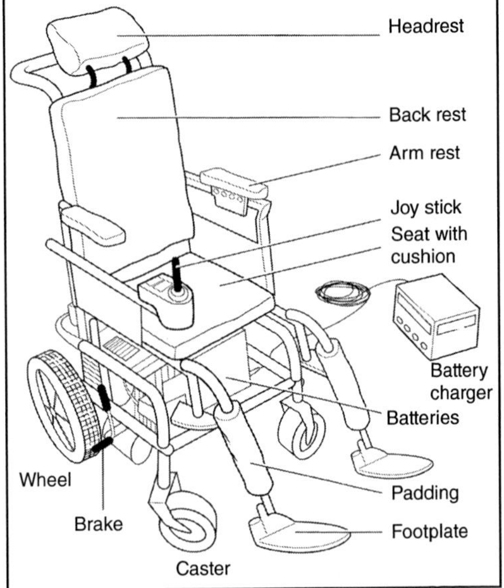

C5 Tetraplegia

- Power wheelchair with power tilt and/or recline
- Modified joystick or head control to operate wheelchair
- Excellent pressure relief seat cushion

- High-back seat, headrest, trunk supports
- Upper extremity support such as lap board, or arm trough

C6 Tetraplegia

Prescribing a wheelchair for a C6 tetraplegic can be challenging. Some individuals may be able to use a manual wheelchair for all activities. Others, due to strength, endurance, cardiovascular fitness or body type, will require a power wheelchair for some community activities. Others may benefit from a power wheelchair for all activities. With aging, pregnancy or musculoskeletal injury (e.g., rotator cuff tendonitis), a person who was initially utilizing a manual wheelchair may now require a power wheelchair.

Power Wheelchairs for C6 Tetraplegia

- Joystick controls
- Power tilt, except if patient is able to consistently perform pressure relief strategies.
  In this case, power tilt is not required.
- Appropriate back height
- Excellent pressure relieving seat cushion

Manual Wheelchairs for C6 Tetraplegia

- Lightweight adjustable manual wheelchair
- Solid back
- Adjustable wheel position
- Modified hand rims (lugs or plastic coated)
- Brake extensions
- Excellent pressure relief cushion

Manual Wheelchairs for C7— T1 Tetraplegia

- Lightweight adjustable manual wheelchair
- Solid back
- Adjustable wheel position
- Modified hand rims (lugs or plastic coated)
- Brake extensions
- Excellent pressure relief seat cushion

Manual Wheelchairs for paraplegic (T2 and below)

- Lightweight adjustable manual wheelchair
- Adjustable wheel position
- Back height may be lowered due to better truncal stability
- Wheels can be placed interiorly for improved maneuverability
- Armrests may not be necessary
- Good pressure relief seat cushion

Seating Systems

Seating systems consist of back supports and cushions (Table 1). These systems should provide proper pressure distribution, enhance truncal and pelvic stability, and provide comfort. Seating systems should be durable and should not retain perspiration or unacceptable odors.

Back supports can be made from a variety of materials. A good back support must be comfortable and should enhance truncal stability. The height of the back support is dependent on truncal stability, amount of spasticity, and level of injury.

Shower Wheelchairs

This is a special type of wheelchair that allows individuals with SCI to roll into a

shower stall. It is generally used by tetraplegics. This type of chair has padded seats and allows access to the perineal areas. High tetraplegics will require a seating system with a high back, as well as tilt and/or recline capability. In addition, arm, neck and head supports may be required.

Power Wheelchair Drive Positions

Wheelchair Drive Position	Potential Positives	Considerations
Rear 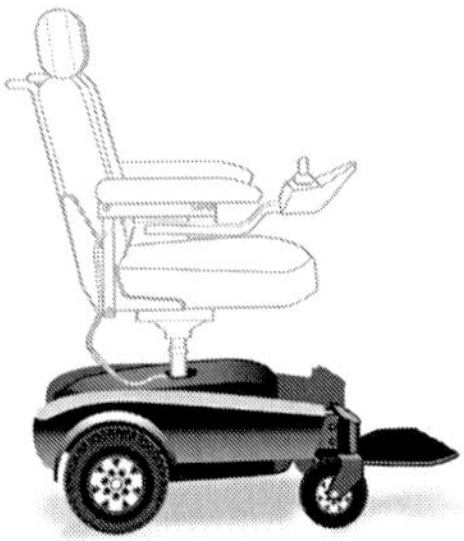	• Good directional control at higher speeds • Stable • Climbs well • Good control with alternate drive controls	• Biggest footprint • Biggest turning radius • Poorer downhill traction on steep slopes • Obstacle climbing might be difficult
Front 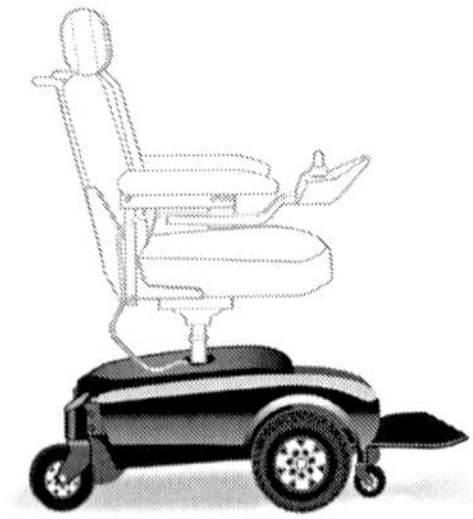	• Climbs obstacles and curbs well • Can position feet at tighter angles	• Limited to slower overall speeds because of poor directional control • Poor directional control – "fishtailing" • Poorer control with non-proportional inputs • Longer turning radius
Mid 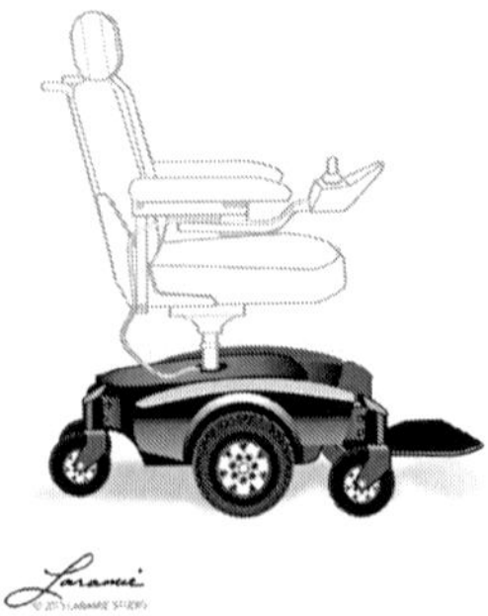	• Intuitive to drive • Small turning radius • Compact design • Transitions well over uneven surfaces if wheels have independent suspension	• Drive wheels will require independent suspension for best climbing and terrain navigation • Needs 6 wheels for stability • Needs some sort of anti-pitch technology to keep base level when climbing or managing uneven terrain

Table 1 Wheelchair Cushion Options

CUSHION TYPE	Pressure Relief	Seating Firmness	Heat Dissipation	Cleanability	Durability	Price
Contoured foam with gel insert 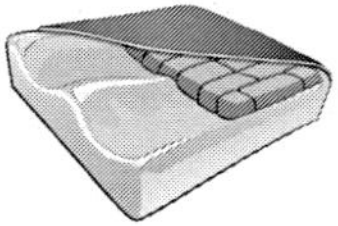	GOOD	GOOD TO EXCELLENT	FAIR TO GOOD	EXCELLENT	GOOD TO EXCELLENT	HIGH
Air-filled villous 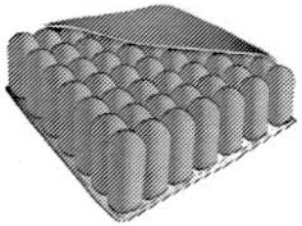	EXCELLENT	POOR TO FAIR	GOOD TO EXCELLENT	EXCELLENT	FAIR TO GOOD	HIGH
Gel-filled 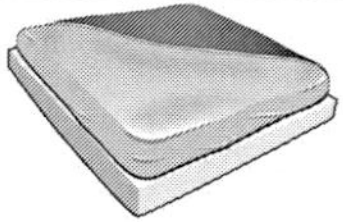	GOOD	FAIR TO GOOD	EXCELLENT	EXCELLENT	FAIR	MODERATE TO HIGH
Coated contoured foam 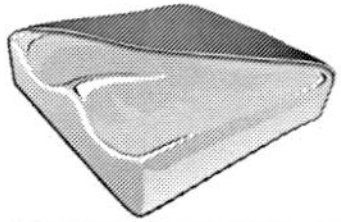	FAIR TO GOOD	EXCELLENT	POOR TO FAIR	EXCELLENT	EXCELLENT	MODERATE TO HIGH
Foam 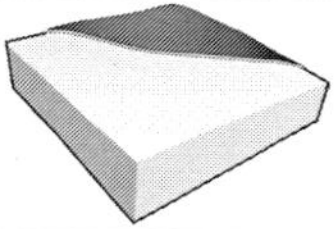	FAIR TO GOOD	GOOD	FAIR	POOR	FAIR TO GOOD	LOW TO MODERATE
Air-filled 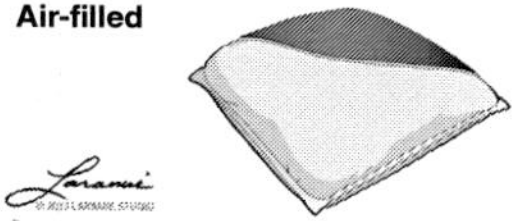	FAIR	GOOD TO EXCELLENT	FAIR TO GOOD	EXCELLENT	GOOD	LOW

Adapted from Kottke FJ, Lehman JF, editors. Krusen's handbook of physical medicine and rehabilitation. 4th ed. Philadelphia: W.B. Saunders; 1990; 560.

Chapter 18

Environmental Modifications

Jim McCormack

Introduction

Securing an accessible apartment or house is a challenge for many persons with SCI. In some communities, the waiting period to obtain a subsidized wheelchair accessible apartment may be greater than one year. Generally, it is easier to obtain an accessible apartment if the injured person is able to pay market rent. Environmental modifications can be expensive and more difficult to perform in communities with older housing stock. If the home is rented, the cooperation of the property owner is required.

Home Modifications

Home modifications are changes to the structure of the home which allow a person with SCI to safely improve access and usability. There are a wide variety of potential home modifications and technologies available for individuals with SCI that are specific to an individual's level of injury. There are, however, some basic principles to understand. Most SCI individuals utilize a wheelchair for mobility. As a result, furniture in the home must be at an accessible height. For example, the cooking surfaces, light switches, and bed surfaces must be placed at a lower height than they are for an able-bodied person. In addition, the wheelchair must be maneuverable throughout the home, which requires wider passageways and low-resistance floors.

The nature and scope of the home modifications and technological interventions required are closely related to the level of injury. Persons with high tetraplegia, who have essentially no upper extremity function, will require the most modifications and devices. These individuals will require an environmental control system that allows for the direction of multiple daily tasks such as opening doors, turning on lights, and operating the stereo. Entrances and hallways must be wide enough to accommodate a large, power wheelchair and possibly a ventilator. Those with mid-level tetraplegia (i.e., C6) with some intact arm function may be able to perform some tasks if appropriate modifications are made. For example, modifying a standard round faucet to a lever-handled faucet may allow for more independent grooming. Individuals with lower-level tetraplegia (i.e., C8) and paraplegia will be able to manipulate objects with their hands. Consequently, fewer environmental modifications will be required.

In some cases, modifications and devices that may improve functional independence cannot be obtained due to funding limitations. Clinicians should be sensitive to budgetary issues and may assist clients in locating creative funding solutions and modification alternatives.

Home modifications of the entrance, kitchen, bathroom and bedroom are critical. They must be undertaken only after close consultation with the person with SCI,

contractor, occupational therapist, physical therapist and physician. It is imperative that reputable, experienced vendors and contractors are selected.

Entrance

A proper, safe entrance is essential. It should be brightly lit so the individual can see keys and locks easily and adequately negotiate any potential irregularities in ground surface. Ideally, the entrance should be covered to offer shelter in inclement weather. If the resident utilizes a van or car, a covered garage or carport is optimal.

Outdoor Elevator

The decision to build an exterior elevator ("porch lift") instead of a ramp must be individualized. If space is limited or the height to traverse is excessive, then an elevator may be the safer choice. If a porch lift is desired, there should be an adequate landing platform (at least 30" x 40"). The control device must be at an accessible height to be usable (e.g., a joystick).

Characteristics of a Ramp

The maximum acceptable slope of a ramp is 1:12 (i.e., one foot of rise for every 12 feet of run). A less severe grade (1:20) will improve accessibility for individuals with limited endurance and upper body strength. The width of the ramp should have a minimum clearance of 36 inches. Landings at the top and bottom of the ramp should be at least 60 inches in length. If the ramp changes direction, the landing should be at least 60 square inches. If the landing is in front of a door, it should be at least 60 square inches. If a ramp has run of more than six feet, it should have handrails on both sides at a height of 32 inches from the ramp surface. It should be noted that, depending on space, these dimensions may need to be modified for private residences.

The door at the end of a ramp should be wide enough to accommodate the individual's wheelchair. An inward door swing is preferred. In addition, the resident should be able to open the door. A person with C7 tetraplegia may require door modifications (i.e., a long-lever, U-handled door), whereas an individual with C4 tetraplegia may require an electronically unlocking and mechanically opening door.

Kitchen

A well-designed kitchen will enhance the independence of a person with an SCI. Reach and maneuvering space are important. Counters and appliances should be placed to allow for the greatest degree of access throughout the kitchen. Clutter exacerbates inaccessibility and should be avoided.

One accessible work space that is at least 30 inches long for food preparation is necessary. It is important to avoid sharp projections or rough surfaces that may abrade insensate skin. Cabinets placed under the counter will be difficult to access for a person in a wheelchair. "Roll-out cabinets" and "Lazy Susan" devices will improve accessibility of stored food items.

Appliance selection should be carefully considered. The controls of ranges and cook tops should be front-mounted to prevent reaching across cooking surfaces. If there is an open area below the cooking surface, it should be well-insulated to prevent burns and electrical shock. Ovens should be self-cleaning and located next to a counter with clear

floor space below it. Side-opening oven doors are desirable. Controls should be on the front of the oven. Refrigerator/freezers should be side-by-side or have at least 50 percent of the freezer space under 54 inches in height and 100 percent of the refrigerator space and the controls under 54 inches. The freezer should be self-defrosting.

Bathroom

The design of the bathroom should accommodate the individual's level of independence. The design should facilitate wheelchair maneuverability, personal grooming, and safe transfers. There should be clear approaches, properly placed grab bars, and non-slip surfaces.

The following should be considered when designing an accessible bathroom:

- To facilitate safe wheelchair-to-commode transfers, the distance between the wall and the center of the toilet seat should be 18 inches. Grab bars should be mounted on at least one side of the toilet. The toilet seat should be between 15 and 16 inches in height. Persons with some ability to stand may benefit from a slightly higher seat (17" to 19"). The toilet paper dispenser should be wall-mounted on the side wall and within easy reach. The dispenser should be installed at a maximum height of 26 inches.
- Sinks should allow for front approach. There should be 29 inches of clearance below the sink, and the minimum depth should be 19 inches. Faucets should be lever, push or electronically controlled.
- The bathing area will depend on the SCI individual's level of injury and functional capabilities. For a person with high tetraplegia, a roll-in shower is most appropriate. If bathing cannot be performed independently, then additional space should be allocated for an attendant. If the person has a lower cervical lesion or paraplegia, a tub bench may be obtained to facilitate safe transfers. A flexible hose and hand-held shower should be installed. To prevent burns, water temperature must be regulated (either at the water heater or with a thermostatic valve). Grab bars should be mounted along two sides.

Bedroom

A firm mattress at a height of 20 to 22 inches is appropriate. There should be three feet between the bed and wall to allow for level, safe transfers. A phone and alarm clock should be placed on a stand or table close to the bed. A roll-in closet with lowered clothing rods may be helpful. A "Closet Carousel" is a mechanical device that will bring items on the clothing rack to the front of the closet. This will increase convenience and accessibility.

Home Automation Devices

Home automation devices (HAD) refer to the wide range of generic environmental control devices that typically control one aspect of the environment. There are thousands of HAD in the marketplace that may assist a person with an SCI to be more independent. Examples include a remote control garage door opener, motion sensing outdoor floodlights, and automatic programmable thermostats. These devices are typically designed for able-bodied people who want to save time, energy or space. HAD sometimes require modifications to assist people with SCI in controlling the home and work environment. Many of these devices can be incorporated into new home and

office construction. There are a few HAD, like motorized counter tops, that are designed specifically for people with disabilities.

Environmental Control Unit

An environmental control unit (ECU) is a tool for purposefully manipulating and interacting with the environment by accessing multiple electrical devices via technological adaptations. Unlike HAD, ECU are developed for and marketed specifically to individuals with disabilities. Each ECU product is designed to allow a person to control numerous aspects of his physical surroundings. Some issues related to selecting an ECU include the number of activities to be directed and cost. In addition, some users will require a portable unit that can be attached to the wheelchair. There are also ECU that are "stand-alone" systems, as well as systems that can be integrated with a home computer.

Two basic questions must be answered prior to purchasing an HAD or ECU. One, what part of the environment does the person want to direct (i.e., turning on lights, operating the telephone)? Two, how can the person operate the controller? Individuals with SCI may use a joystick, chin controls, sip-and-puff controls, or voice controls. Technology currently exists that allows a person to control most aspects of his environment with any part of the body capable of consistent movement. Even if this movement is minimal (e.g., the chin), the ECU can capitalize on this ability for optimal environmental control.

The manner of control (how a device is activated) is a critical consideration in the selection of ECU and HAD. The basic methods of control include direct wire, infrared, radio frequency and power line. The direct wire method involves directly wiring an adapted switch or controller to the device to be controlled. Infrared control is built into many electronic appliances, such as a television remote, and requires a clear line of sight between the controller and the device being controlled. Radio frequency control offers wireless control without the line of sight requirement. Power line control uses a combination of controllers and modules that plug into standard office or home AC outlets. On/off signals are sent from each controller to the device to be controlled via standard AC wiring. Unlike direct wire control, no additional wiring or modification is required with power line control systems.

Home modifications and technological devices can improve the quality of life for persons with SCI. These can be expensive, however, and must be prescribed judiciously. It is also imperative that the person with SCI be involved in the selection and provision of any device or intervention.

Chapter 19

Community Reintegration in the American Context

*Allan R. Meyers**
Andrew Graham

The ultimate goal of the rehabilitation process is to reintegrate an individual with SCI into the community. The level of participation in family, vocational, avocational and civic activities is influenced by the severity of impairment (i.e., level of injury) and presence of secondary conditions (e.g., traumatic brain injury, pressure ulcer). In addition, the magnitude of financial resources, level of family supports, and scope of psychological adjustment are important. Educational and professional achievement prior to acquiring an SCI also influences community reintegration. Successful reintegration requires interventions on an individual and societal basis. For example, many people with SCI require home modifications to improve accessibility. As many people with SCI do not have the financial resources to pay for these renovations, society must provide the funds (i.e., government, foundations, charity). Furthermore, the community as a whole must have the political will to expend the financial resources to build and maintain architecturally accessible public spaces and transportation.

Community resources and assistance programs vary widely due to differing funding paradigms and eligibility criteria. As such, there is no one prescription or formula to achieve successful reintegration. Physicians must work closely with other professional colleagues (nurses, therapists, social workers and, on occasion, attorneys) as well as with the patient and his friends and family to obtain the appropriate services. This chapter will briefly address some of the issues related to reintegration.

Independent Living Centers

Independent living centers (ILC) in the United States are federally-supported, not-for-profit, consumer-governed organizations for persons with disabilities. ILC are funded at the federal level by the U.S. Department of Education's Rehabilitation Services Administration. Other financial support is derived from state and local governments, as well as by private foundations and individuals. By statute, 50 percent of the boards of directors and employees of ILC must be persons with disabilities. The four core services provided by ILC are information and referral, skills training, peer counseling and advocacy. ILC are excellent resources for identifying and accessing community services. These centers should be contacted during the acute phase of SCI.

*Deceased

Income Support

As noted in chapter 1, many people with SCI were injured at a relatively young age. Many individuals had not completed their vocational training or education, or were at the beginning of their careers at the time of injury. These factors compound the challenges of obtaining paid employment. In addition, as stated in chapter 14, there are significant financial disincentives to remunerated employment.

It is estimated that 75 percent of persons with SCI are not employed; many receive income derived from public and/or private sources. Private income support is primarily in the form of commercial disability insurance benefits and, on occasion, pension benefits (i.e., the individual is "medically retired"). Some individuals may receive the proceeds of legal settlements in either structured settlements or trust income. Others receive Social Security Disability Insurance (SSDI) benefits or Supplemental Social Security Insurance (SSI) benefits. Typically, SSDI benefits are available to those who have contributed to the Social Security program for five of the past 10 years prior to injury. People with SCI should apply for SSDI as early as possible. The benefits are based on the amount of previous contributions and can be supplemented by other private income support programs or family earnings.

If an SSDI recipient returns to paid employment, a part or all of the SSDI benefits may be eliminated. Social Security regulations have promulgated rules regarding returning to work for SSDI recipients. The Social Security Administration (SSA) permits individuals who are receiving SSDI benefits to engage in a "trial work period" for nine months and continue to receive their full SSDI benefits, as well as Medicare insurance coverage. The purpose of the trial work period is to test the recipient's ability to work without losing their benefits or health insurance. The trial work period does not have to be for nine consecutive months. There is an earnings threshold ($750.00 per month for 2013) before the SSA considers that an individual is engaging in substantial gainful employment.

Different rules apply for individuals who are receiving SSI benefits. There is no provision allowing SSI recipients to work for a trial work period, but these individuals may be eligible for special cash benefits and the continuation of their Medicaid coverage if their gross income exceeds the amount defined as substantial gainful employment.

Medical Benefits

In the US, medical benefits are provided by public and private organizations (both for- and not-for-profit). People with SCI may secure benefits through private insurance, Medicaid and Medicare, or a combination of the three.

Private medical insurance is related to employment status, and many times the cost of premiums is partially subsidized by the employer. Of note, only a minority of persons with SCI are employed and, thereby, eligible for private coverage.

Medicaid

Medicaid is a state-administered medical insurance program that is primarily designed for indigent people. Funding is shared by state and federal governments and is based on a complex reimbursement formula. The breadth of services covered, level of financial reimbursement to providers, and financial eligibility criterion vary from state to state. Some states, such as Massachusetts, have relatively comprehensive coverage

that includes durable medical equipment, consumable medical supplies, and personal assistant services. Other Medicaid programs have very limited benefits.

Medicare

Medicare is a federally-funded program. Beneficiaries include older adults (over age 65) and individuals with end-stage renal disease. Disabled persons who are unable to work permanently or for prolonged periods of time may also be eligible.

Medicare consists of Part A (Hospital Benefits), Part B (Traditional Medicare), Part C (Medicare Advantage Plans), and Part D (Prescription Drug Plans). Beneficiaries must decide whether they want to enroll in Medicare Part A and the traditional Part B benefits or if a managed care plan (Part C) is a better option for them, depending upon their medical needs.

Part A does not require any premium payment and pays for inpatient hospital care, skilled nursing home services, hospice care, and home health services. The benefits are subject to co-insurance and deductibles. Part B covers most inpatient or outpatient clinician charges and outpatient diagnostic services. Part B requires the payment of a premium, which generally increases each year.

In general, individuals who are eligible to receive SSDI benefits are eligible for Medicare benefits after a two-year waiting period. In the meantime, persons with SCI have to purchase relatively expensive private health insurance, secure Medicaid benefits, or forgo medical coverage. Some states pay for Part B benefits through the Medicaid program for those with minimal financial resources. In addition, some state Medicaid programs provide reimbursement for co-insurance and deductibles for the profoundly indigent.

In lieu of traditional Medicare, beneficiaries may chose Medicare Part C coverage, which combines Parts A and B and covers all medically needed services. Many managed care insurance programs limit choice in physicians, hospitals and other health-care providers to contain costs. Although enrolled providers in a managed care program may provide adequate choice and expertise for the otherwise well population, these restrictions can be problematic for persons with SCI. Persons with SCI have a unique set of medical issues that may not be adequately addressed by clinicians inexperienced in SCI care.

Durable Medical Equipment and Consumable Supplies

Many private and public insurance carriers place strict (and sometimes unreasonable) restrictions on the provision of durable medical equipment (e.g., wheelchairs, tub benches, etc.). Obtaining coverage for consumable medical supplies, such as urinary catheters and latex gloves, may also be difficult.

Veterans Benefits

The Department of Veterans Affairs (VA) operates a national network of hospitals and clinics that care for persons with SCI. VA services are available to all veterans who have served a minimum of 24 months on active duty and have been honorably discharged. VA benefits are also available to those individuals who suffered an SCI due to a service-related injury (e.g., a wartime gunshot wound). Veterans may be eligible

for a relatively unknown program called Aid and Attendance Benefits. The program has several benefits that may be particularly helpful to individuals with SCI.

Affordable Care Act

Beginning on January 1, 2014, the Patient Protection and Affordable Care Act mandates that every person in the US must be covered under a health insurance plan. States may establish their own "insurance exchange programs" or allow the federal government to do so, allowing individuals to shop for individual private insurance plans. The Act also expands eligibility for Medicaid coverage, including coverage for low-income people who do not have children. The federal government will fund coverage for these newly eligible adults. For those who cannot afford to purchase private health insurance and are eligible for Medicaid, the federal government also offers subsidies to expand Medicaid benefits. The governors of several states, however, have indicated that they will not set up insurance exchange programs in their states, despite funding from the federal government, and it is unclear how the Affordable Care Act will impact the Medicaid program.

Personal Assistant Services

Many persons with SCI require others to assist with basic personal care needs such as bathing, grooming, dressing and toileting, as well as light household tasks such as cooking and cleaning. In some cases, family members provide these services without remuneration. However, the provision of these services may distort and potentially strain family relationships.

Personal assistant services can be provided by paid personal care assistants (PCA). These services are essential for persons with SCI to live in the community, and can be provided by licensed or unlicensed individuals. In keeping with the independent living philosophy, PCA care must be directed by the person with SCI. Historically, the employer-employee relationship has been between the disabled person and the PCA. However, there are some regulatory burdens associated with employer status (e.g., withholding taxes, paying workers' compensation insurance, etc.). As such, some states may provide alternate payment paradigms. For example, the state or a financial intermediary may become the employer of record and assume responsibility for compliance with appropriate employment statutes.

PCA services may be reimbursed by state Medicaid programs, workers' compensation benefits, or proceeds from legal settlements. In general, private insurance carriers do not pay for PCA services. On occasion, disabled individuals may pay for services from their own financial resources. In addition, some persons with SCI provide non-cash benefits to PCAs such as free room and board.

Public Transportation

Federal and state legislation mandates accessible public bus and rail transportation. These directives, however, have not been fully implemented, and it is still challenging for a person with SCI to travel on local and regional transit systems.

Para-transit is an alternative form of public transportation. Typically, vans equipped with hydraulic lifts provide door-to-door transportation at a modest cost. To utilize services, an individual must provide some medical documentation to demonstrate

eligibility. Some para-transit systems (but not all) may allow a PCA and small children to accompany the disabled person. Para-transit services may, on occasion, prioritize requests for transportation; for example, medical appointments may supersede recreational visits, and patrons who had scheduled trips may be "bumped" to provide transportation for other disabled persons.

Private transportation may be the best alternative. Lower-level tetraplegics and paraplegics should be able to drive an appropriately chosen and properly modified automobile. Many higher level tetraplegics may operate a specially modified van. The cost of a customized vehicle, however, may range from $35,000 to $50,000. Although private transportation can improve quality of life for a person with SCI, finding adequate funding remains a significant challenge.

Chapter 20

Community Reintegration in the Canadian Context

Adriano Persi

Medical Benefits

In Canada, there is a publicly-funded health-care system that provides a comprehensive array of clinical services. These services are available to every legal resident. The public system is administered by the provincial governments via the Ministry of Health or similar entity, but is funded by the provincial and federal governments. There is some variability in the scope and availability of services across provinces. Typically, the cost of acute hospitalization, inpatient rehabilitation, and most physician services are provided without cost to people with spinal cord injury (SCI). More variably, most provinces have publicly-funded programs to assist people with SCI obtain consumable medical supplies and durable medical equipment; many times, a co-payment by the beneficiary is required. A subset of patients may have access to supplemental resources, such as employer-funded benefit plans, depending on their specific circumstances.

It should be noted, however, that in Canada a number of important health-care services are typically not completely publicly funded. The level of funding, if any, varies among the provinces. Potentially unfunded services include prescription eyeglasses, outpatient physical therapy, and occupational therapy, as well as dental, podiatry, chiropractic and optometric services. In most cases, patients over the age of 65 receive prescription medications at a reduced cost from provincial programs. However, people with limited financial resources may access some of these services through social welfare programs. The most commonly covered service is prescription drug benefits.

In addition to provincial health-care programs, these are other entities that provide financial support for health-care services for people with SCI. Members of the National Defense Forces, Royal Canadian Mounted Police, or the Canadian Security Intelligence Services receive health-care services through their respective public employer. For those who experience a work-related SCI, medical benefits and income support are available from their respective provincial workers' compensation boards. For those who experience a motor vehicle accident related to SCI, financial support for health-care services may be supplemented by benefits from the automobile insurance system. This may include funding directly from the insurance carrier and/or the proceeds of a tort claim.

Income Support

People with SCI may be eligible for any number of supports. Canadian Pension Plan (CPP) disability benefits are part of a federally-administered public social insurance

system. Employees and employers are required to make contributions based on earned income. Benefits are contingent on the amount of contributions and the length of plan membership. In addition, there are provincially-funded and -administered disability income support programs. The only significant consideration for eligibility is to meet residency requirements, which vary by province.

Some individuals, such as members of the military, may also be eligible for service-related pensions. Furthermore, workers' compensation benefits may be a source of income support for a work-related SCI. However, not all workers are covered by workers' compensation programs. Some people with SCI also are covered by private (self- or employer-funded) disability income support. If the SCI was related to a motor vehicle collision, income support may be provided by the insurance carrier as a "no-fault" benefit. Some patients may secure income support legal settlements related to tort action; these funds may be provided in a single payment ("lump sum") or, alternatively, as a structured settlement with guaranteed annuity payments.

Transportation

Public transportation for people with SCI may be available through Disabled & Aged Regional Transportation (DART) services. These services are typically supported by the provincial government and local communities. As this is a community-specific resource, the general availability and level of DART services varies considerably. For example, the eligibility criterion varies from community to community. DART services are more available in urban and suburban areas. Furthermore, as these are community-specific resources, DART services generally do not cross community boundaries. This is problematic for those who need to access services in nearby and neighboring communities.

Many people with SCI are able to drive a modified car or van. The cost of modifications and maintenance is typically borne by the person with SCI. Charitable agencies or service clubs may be available to some to provide financial support for the modifications.

Conclusion

In 1990, the US Congress passed the landmark Americans with Disabilities Act (ADA). The ADA is emblematic of a worldwide cultural shift; over the past 30 years, similar statutes have been passed by jurisdictions throughout the world. The overall societal imperative is to enable and encourage people with disabilities to fully participate in the opportunities and challenges of an inclusive society.

Treating a person with SCI is an excellent case study of the rehabilitation process. When intially admitted to the hospital, the patient passively receives the care and treatment of medical, nursing and allied health professionals. As the individual progresses and is transferred to the rehabilitation unit, the injured person is encouraged to depend on his own capabilities or to effectively direct the care provided by others. Finally, with community reintegration, the injured individual is less of a patient and more of a consumer of medical, social and community services.

Typically, people with SCI are living three and four decades from their original injury. However, as consumers of health-care resources, it is important that people with SCI engage their clinicians, caregivers and families in a dialogue about issues related to life-sustaining technologies and end-of-life care. There is no prescriptive answer to what technology and life-sustaining services a patient may request. This may be an uncomfortable dialogue. Ideally, this is a discussion that should be initiated at a time when a person is well and not under pressure due to imminent hospitalization and/or illness.

Advances in knowledge and technology have improved the ability of clinicians to diagnose and treat people with SCI. In addition, research has expanded understanding of the pathophysiology of SCI. Collectively, this has contributed to people with SCI reaching higher levels of physical function and social participation. Nevertheless, many issues related to SCI have not been studied in a rigorous scientific manner. The contributors hope that this monograph will, in some small way, inspire researchers and caregivers of people with SCI to continue expanding the biological and sociomedical understanding of SCI.

Appendix 1–Suggested Readings

Chapter 1

Devivo MJ. Epidemiology of traumatic spinal cord injury: trends and future implications. Spinal Cord 2012; 50(5): 365-72.

Cripps RA, Lee BB, Wing P, et al. A global map for traumatic spinal cord injury epidemiology: towards a living data repository for injury prevention. Spinal Cord 2011; 49(4): 493-501.

Spinal Cord Injury Model System Information Network: http://www.uab.edu/medicine_sci

Noonan VK, Fingas M, Farry A, et al. Incidence and prevalence of spinal cord injury in Canada: a national perspective. Neuroepidemiology 2012; 38(4); 219-26.

Pickett GE, Campos-Benitez M, Keller JL, et al. Epidemiology of traumatic spinal cord injury in Canada. Spine (Phila, PA 1976) 2006; 31(7): 799-805.

Couris CM, Guilcher SJ, Munce SE, et al. Characteristics of adults with incident traumatic spinal cord injury in Ontario, Canada. Spinal Cord 2010; 48: 39-44.

Dryden DM, Saunders LD, Rowe BH, et al. The epidemiology of traumatic spinal cord injury in Alberta, Canada. Can J Neurol Sci 2003; 30(2): 113-21.

Chapter 2

Kakulas BA. Neuropathology: the foundation for new treatments in spinal cord injury. Spinal Cord 2004; 42: 549-63.

Chapter 3

Bracken MB, Shepard MJ, Collins WF, et al. A randomized controlled trial of methylprednisolone or naloxone in the treatment of acute spinal cord injury. N Eng J Med 1990; 322: 1405-11.

Bracken MB, Shepard MJ, Holford TR, et al. Administration of methylprednisolone for 24 or 48 hours or tirilazad mesylate for 48 hours in the treatment of acute spinal cord injury. J Am Med Assoc 1997; 277: 1597-1604.

Nesathurai S. Steroids and spinal cord injury: revisiting NASCIS 2 and NASCIS 3 trials. J Trauma 1998; 1088-93.

Geisler FH, Dorsey FC, Coleman WP. Recovery of motor function after spinal cord injury: a randomized, placebo-controlled trial with GM-1 ganglioside. N Eng J Med 1997; 324(26): 1829-38.

Bagnall AM, Jones L, Duffy S, et al. Spinal fixation surgery for acute traumatic spinal cord injury. Cochrane Database Syst Rev 2008; (1): CD004725.

Chapter 4

Waring P, Biering-Sorenson F, Burns SP, et al. 2009 review and revisions of the international standards for the neurological classification of spinal cord injury. J Spinal Cord Med 2010; 33(4): 346-52.

American Spinal Cord Injury Association. International Standards for Neurological Classification of Spinal Cord Injury, revised 2000; Atlanta, reprinted 2008.

American Spinal Cord Injury Association. Reference Manual for the International Standards for Neurological Classification of Spinal Cord Injury. Chicago, 2003.

Kirshblum SC, Burns SP, Biering-Sorenson F, et al. International standards for neurological classification of spinal cord injury (revised 2011). J Spinal Cord Med 2011; 34(6): 535-46.

Frankel HL, Hancock DO, Hyslop G, et al. The value of postural reduction in the initial management of closed injuries in the spine with paraplegia and tetraplegia. Paraplegia 1969; 7(3): 179-92.

Kirshblum SC, Waring WP, Biering-Sorenson F, et al. Reference for the 2011 revision of the international standards for neurological classification of spinal cord injury. J Spinal Cord Med 2011; 34(6): 457-54.

American Spinal Injury Association ASIA Learning Center. www.asialearningcenter.com

Chapter 5

Paralyzed Veterans of America. Outcomes Following Traumatic Spinal Cord Injury. Washington, DC.

Paralyzed Veterans of America. Preservation of Upper Limb Function Following Spinal Cord injury. Washington, DC.

Chapter 6

Paralyzed Veterans of America. Early Acute Management in Adults with Spinal Cord Injury. Washington, DC.

Chapter 7

Paralyzed Veterans of America. Bladder Management for Adults with Spinal Cord Injury. Washington, DC.

Chapter 8

Paralyzed Veterans of America. Neurogenic Bowel Management in Adults with Spinal Cord Injury. Washington, DC.

Chapter 9

Paralyzed Veterans of America. Pressure Ulcer Prevention and Treatment Following Spinal Cord Injury. Washington, DC.

Chapter 10

Yarkony GM. Contractures complicating spinal cord injury: incidence and comparison between spinal cord center and general hospital acute care. Paraplegia 1985; 23: 265-71.

Halar E, Bell K. Contracture and other deleterious effects of immobility. In: DeLisa J, editor: Rehabilitation Medicine Principles and Practice. Philadelphia: 1988; 448-55.

Chapter 11

Banister R, Matias C, eds. Autonomic Failure: A Textbook of Clinical Disorders of the Autonomic Nervous System. Third edition. Oxford University Press; 1992; 839-81.

Braddon RL, Rocco JF. Autonomic dysreflexia: a survey of current treatment. Am J Phys Med Rehab 1991: 70: 234-41.

Colachis SC III. Autnomic hyperreflexia with spinal cord injury. J Am Paraplegia Soc 1992; 15: 171-86.

Autonomic dysreflexia in spinal cord injury. http://emedicine.medscape.com/article/322809-overview

National Spinal Cord Injury Association. www.spinalcord.org/resource-center/askus/index.php?pg=kb.page&id-1394

Chapter 12

Brashear A, Elovic E. (2010) Spasticity: Diagnosis and Management. New York: Demos Medical Publishing.

Chapter 13

Baldwin K, Namdari S, Hosalkar H, et al. What's new in orthopedic rehabilitation. J Bone Joint Surg (AM) 2012; 94A(22): 2106-11.

Chapter 14

Paralyzed Veterans of America. Depression Following Spinal Cord Injury. Washington, DC.

Chapter 15

Paralyzed Veterans of America. Sexuality and Reproductive Health in Adults with Spinal Cord Injury. Washington, DC.

Ducharme SH, Gill KM. (1997) Sexuality after Spinal Cord Injury. Baltimore, MD: Paul Brookes Publishing Co.

Chapter 16

Paralyzed Veterans of America. Respiratory Management Following Spinal Cord Injury. Washington, DC.

Chapter 17

Croteau C. Wheelchair Mobility. Worcester, MA: Park Press Publishing; 1998.

Chapter 18

Eberhardt KE. Home modifications for persons with spinal cord injury. OT Practice, 3(10): 24-7.

Salmen JP. The do able renewable home. Washington: American Association of Retired Persons.

Chapter 19

Scelza WM, Kirshblum SC, Wuermser LA, et al. Community reintegration after spinal cord injury. Arch Phys Med Rehabil 2007; 88(3 Suppl 1): S71-5.

Oh DW, Park HJ. One-year follow-up of the effects of community-based ambulation training for ambulatory patients with incomplete spinal cord injury: a case series. NeuroRehabilitation 2013; 32(2): 425-32.

Chapter 20

Canada Pension Plan Disability Programs. www.servicecanada.gc.ca/eng/isp/cpp/partners.shtml

Department of Veterans Affairs. www.veterans.gc.ca/eng/services

Canadian Home Care Association. www.cdnhomecare.ca

Canadian Home Care Association Health Systems Integration Synthesis Report. www.cdnhomecare.ca/media.php?mid=2965

Index

Tables

Illustrations

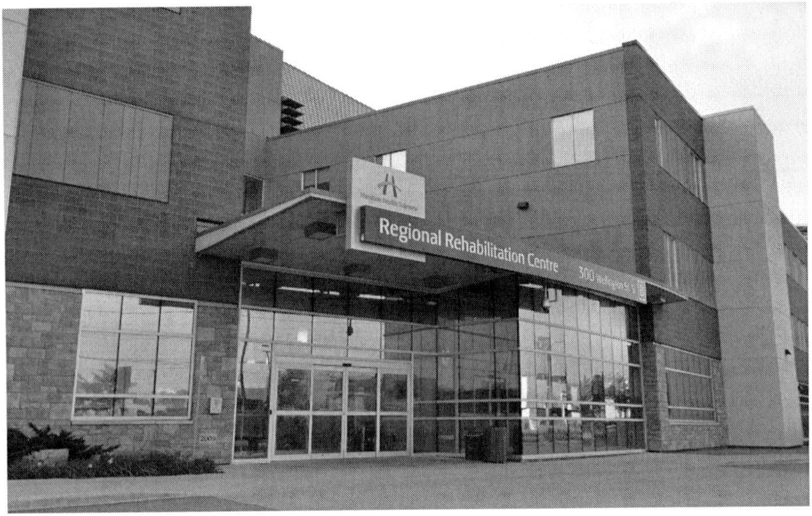

Hamilton Health Sciences

Hamilton Health Sciences, a group of hospitals in Hamilton, Ontario, is a major teaching affiliate of McMaster University School of Medicine. This academic medical center includes the following campuses: Hamilton General Hospital, Juravinski Cancer Center, Juravinski Hospital, McMaster University Medical Center, McMaster Children's Hospital, and St. Peter's Hospital.

With approximately 1,200 beds, Hamilton Health Sciences is the second largest health system in Canada and the regional referral center for nearly 2.3 million people. The hospital group provides acute medical and surgical services, as well as acute and subacute rehabilitation programs.

Hamilton Health Sciences has been providing inpatient and outpatient rehabilitation care for more than 75 years. The Department of Physical Medicine and Rehabilitation supports approximately 150 acute rehabilitation beds, which are co-located on the campuses of the acute care hospitals. Specialized rehabilitation programs treat people with spinal cord injury, traumatic brain injury, orthopedic conditions, and cancer. Its large prosthetics and orthotics program includes an in-house manufacturing facility. The department also supports one of the largest residency training programs in Canada.

Essentials of Inpatient Rehabilitation

Shanker Nesathurai, MD, FRCP(C)
David Blaustein, MD
Editors

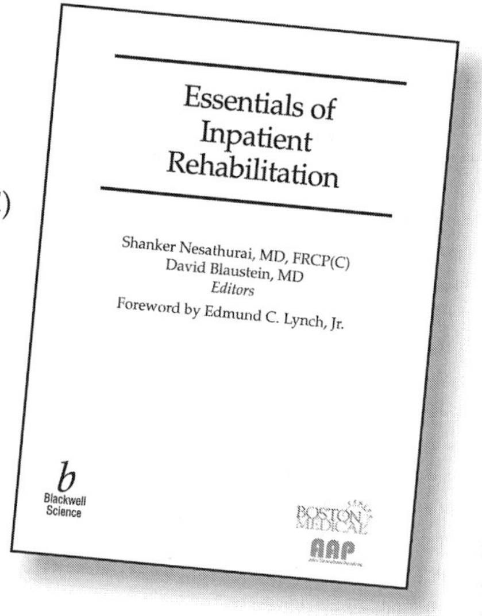

The Essentials of Inpatient Rehabilitation is a concise monograph that reviews the major clinical disorders managed in an acute rehabilitation venue. Topics covered include total joint replacement, fracture, stroke, multiple sclerosis, amputation, and peripheral vascular disease. There is a discussion of fundamental concepts such as the organization of rehabilitation programs, indications for therapeutic exercise, and the rationale for passive interventions. This monograph contains 142 pages and 18 original illustrations.

To order: Arbuckle Academic Publishing
82 Fairlawn Street
Whitinsville, MA 01588
Tel: 508-234-4494
Email: arbuckleacademicpub@gmail.com
$25, plus shipping

For the Pastor-counselor's reference or to lend to others:

Why Wait till Marriage? by Dr. Isabelo F. Magalit
Love and Courtship by Evelyn Miranda-Feliciano
To Have and to Hold by William B. Girao
Ten Commandments for Husbands and Wives by Dr. Harold J. Sala
Life and Love (a Christian view of sex) by Dr. Clyde Narramore
Living Joyfully as a Single in a Couples' World by Dr. Harold J. Sala
The Bondage Breaker by Neil T. Anderson
Being Single Is Better Than Being Married To An Unsuitable Partner by William B. Girao
Coffee Cup Counseling by Dr. Harold J. Sala
Coping with Stress by Dr. Harold J. Sala
Counterfeit by Donald Platt
*Exercising Leadership in the Local Church** by William B. Girao
Family Planning: Theological, Medical and Legal Perspectives edited by Dr. Isabelo F. Magalit
*Filipino Values and Our Christian Faith** by Evelyn Miranda-Feliciano
Filipino Spirit World by Rodney L. Henry
Finding God's Will by Zac Poonen
Helping People Step Out of Homosexuality by Frank Worthen
How to Have a Healing Ministry in Any Church by C. Peter Wagner
More Than Love by Will and Jacquie Chevalier
The Act of Marriage by Tim and Beverly LaHaye
How to Win Over Worry by John Haggai
The Renewed Mind by Larry Christenson
Restoring the Fallen by Drs. Isabelo F. Magalit and Josue D. Ganibe
What Cancer Cannot Do by E.S. Leung
Winning Your Inner Struggles by Dr. Harold J. Sala

* Filipino translation available

9/2M/6.2000